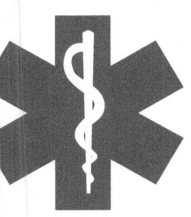

Trauma Case Studies for the Paramedic

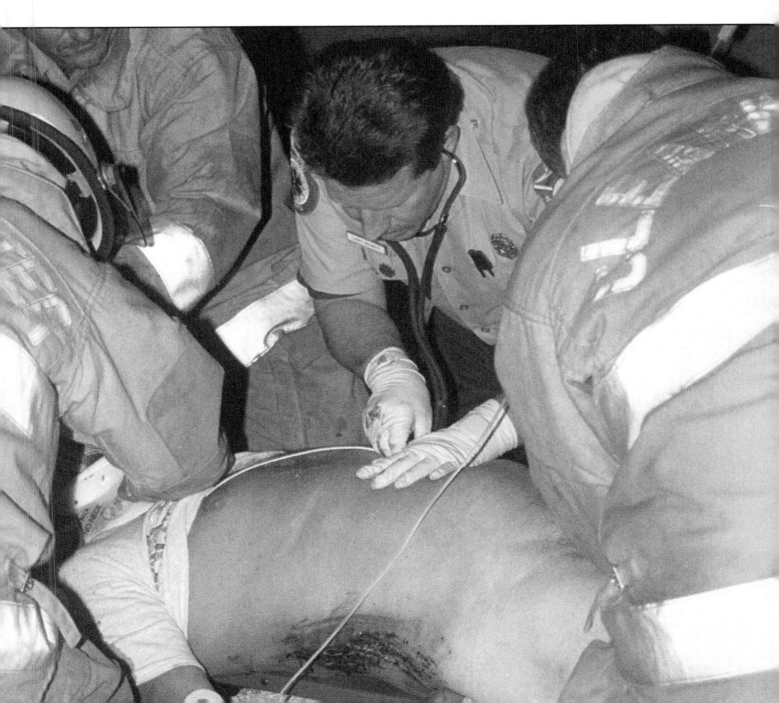

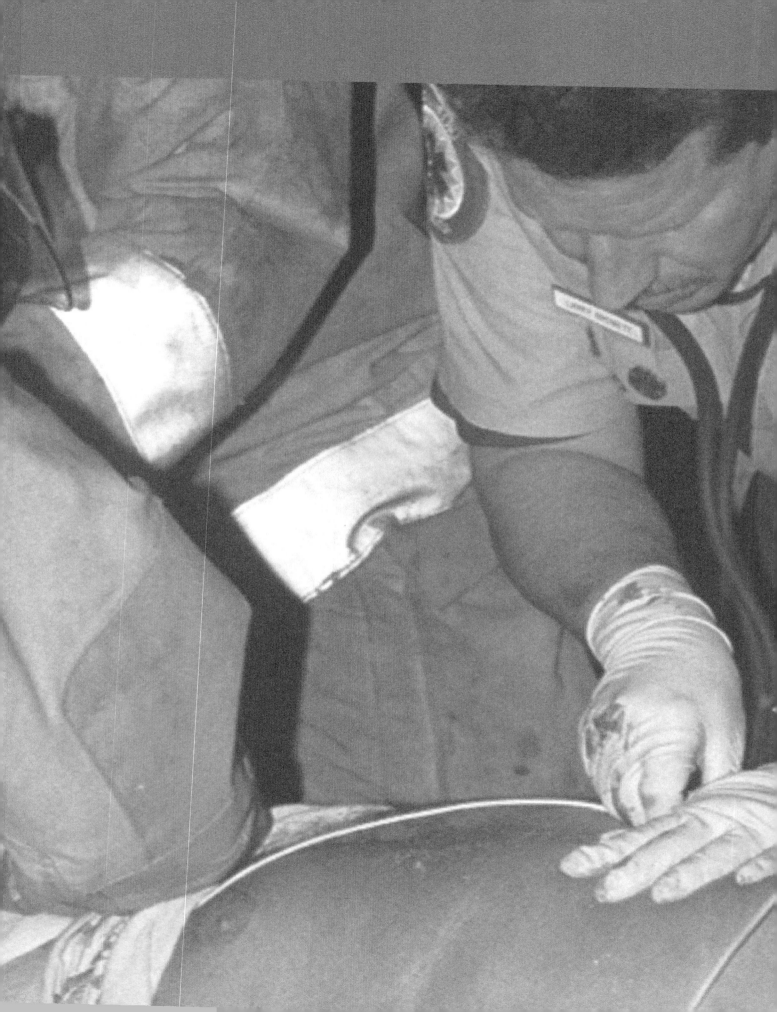

AAOS

Trauma Case Studies for the Paramedic

Stephen J. Rahm, NREMT-P
Author
Kendall County EMS Training Institute
Boerne, Texas

Andrew N. Pollak, MD, EMT-P, FAAOS
Medical Editor
University of Maryland School of Medicine
Baltimore County Fire Department
Baltimore, Maryland

JONES AND BARTLETT PUBLISHERS
Sudbury, Massachusetts
BOSTON   TORONTO   LONDON   SINGAPORE

Jones and Bartlett Publishers

World Headquarters
40 Tall Pine Drive
Sudbury, MA 01776
978-443-5000
info@jbpub.com
www.jbpub.com

Jones and Bartlett Publishers Canada
2406 Nikanna Rd.
Mississauga, ON L5C 2W6
Canada

Jones and Bartlett Publishers International
Barb House, Barb Mews
London W6 7PA
United Kingdom

Production Credits
Chief Executive Officer: Clayton Jones
Chief Operating Officer: Donald W. Jones, Jr.
President, Jones and Barlett Higher Education
and Professional Publishing: Robert W. Holland, Jr.
V.P., Design and Production: Anne Spencer
V.P., Sales and Marketing: William Kane
V.P., Manufacturing and Inventory Control: Therese Bräuer
Publisher, Public Safety Group: Kimberly Brophy
Associate Managing Editor: Jennifer Reed
Associate Production Editor: Jenny McIsaac
Director of Marketing: Alisha Weisman
Photo Researcher: Kimberly Potvin
Cover and Text Design: Anne Spencer
Composition: Jason Miranda
Printing and Binding: Courier Stoughton

American Academy of Orthopaedic Surgeons

Editorial Credits
Chief Education Officer: Mark W. Wieting
Director, Department of Publications: Marilyn L. Fox, PhD
Managing Editor: Lynne Roby Shindoll
Senior Editor: Barbara A. Scotese

Photo Credits
Cover Photo © Eddie Sperling
Chapter 6 Opener © Eddie Sperling
Chapter 8 Opener © Eddie Sperling
Chapter 12 Opener Marilyn Westlake
Figure 12-2 © Visuals Unlimited

ISBN: 0-7637-2583-8

Library of Congress Cataloging-in-Publication Data

Rahm, Stephen J.
   Trauma case studies for the paramedic / Stephen Rahm.
      p. ; cm.
   ISBN 0-7637-2583-8 (pbk.)
1. Wounds and injuries—Case studies. 2. Medical emergencies—Case studies.
   [DNLM: 1. Wounds and Injuries—therapy—Case Reports. 2. Wounds and Injuries—therapy—Problems and Exercises. 3. Emergency Medical Services—Case Reports. 4. Emergency Medical Services—Problems and Exercises. 5. Emergency Medical Technicians. 6. Life Support Care—Case Reports. 7. Life Support Care—Problems and Exercises. WO 18.2 R147t 2005] I. Title.
   RC86.7.R336 2005
   617.1—dc22

                                    2004011521

CONTENTS

Review of Trauma Shock xi

Preface xvii

Case Study 1: 47-Year-Old Male Struck with a Steel Pipe 1
    Case Study 1: Answers and Summary 6

Case Study 2: 30-Year-Old Male with Severe Head Trauma 11
    Case Study 2: Answers and Summary 16

Case Study 3: 22-Year-Old Male with a Gunshot Wound to the Chest 23
    Case Study 3: Answers and Summary 28

Case Study 4: 40-Year-Old Male Who Was the Victim of an Assault 35
    Case Study 4: Answers and Summary 40

Case Study 5: 39-Year-Old Male Injured in a House Fire 45
    Case Study 5: Answers and Summary 49

Case Study 6: 50-Year-Old Male with Multiple Injuries 55
    Case Study 6: Answers and Summary 59

Case Study 7: 30-Year-Old Female with Spinal Trauma 63
    Case Study 7: Answers and Summary 67

Case Study 8: 41-Year-Old Male with Traumatic Cardiac Arrest 73
    Case Study 8: Answers and Summary 77

Case Study 9: 19-Year-Old Female with a Fractured Wrist 83
    Case Study 9: Answers and Summary 87

Case Study 10: 37-Year-Old Male with a Stab Wound 91
    Case Study 10: Answers and Summary 96

Case Study 11: 31-Year-Old Female's Passenger Is Killed in a Car Crash 103
    Case Study 11: Answers and Summary 107

Case Study 12: 70-Year-Old Female with a Hip Fracture 111
    Case Study 12: Answers and Summary 115

Case Study 13: 32-Year-Old Pregnant Female Involved in a Car Crash 123
    Case Study 13: Answers and Summary 127

Case Study 14: 18-Year-Old Male Near-Drowning Victim 133
    Case Study 14: Answers and Summary 137

Case Study 15: 25-Year-Old Male with Severe Maxillofacial Trauma 143
    Case Study 15: Answers and Summary 147

Case Study 16: 20-Year-Old Male Who Fell from a Cliff 151
    Case Study 16: Answers and Summary 155

Case Study 17: 44-Year-Old Male with an Open Abdominal Wound 161
    Case Study 17: Answers and Summary 165

Case Study 18: 20-Year-Old Male with a Shoulder Injury 171
    Case Study 18: Answers and Summary 175

Case Study 19: 50-Year-Old Male with Severe External Bleeding 181
    Case Study 19: Answers and Summary 185

Case Study 20: A Mass-Casualty Incident 193
    Case Study 20: Answers and Summary 196

CHAPTER PREVIEW

Text Resources

Trauma Case Studies for the Paramedic contains 20 case studies representing a variety of trauma emergencies. Each case study follows a logical and systematic approach to patient assessment and management. Paramedic students apply knowledge from initial training to real-life scenarios as they complete the case studies and answer corresponding questions.

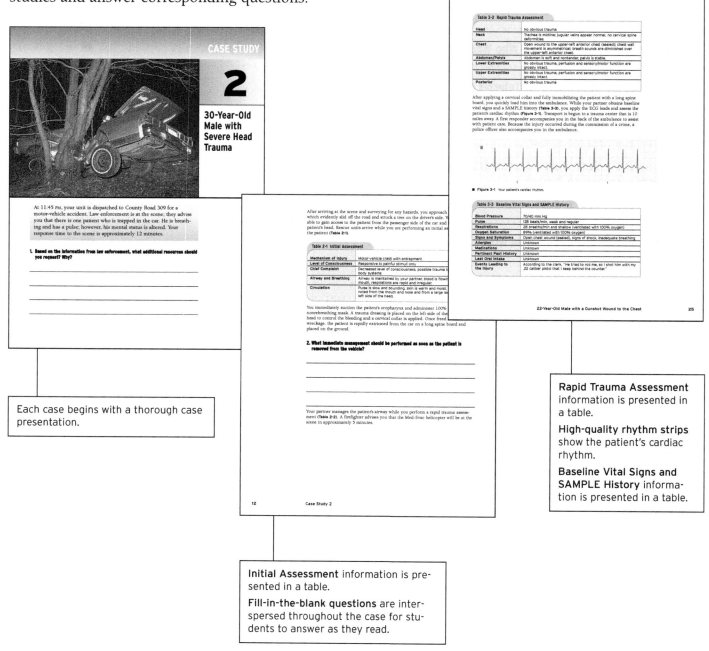

Each case begins with a thorough case presentation.

Rapid Trauma Assessment information is presented in a table.

High-quality rhythm strips show the patient's cardiac rhythm.

Baseline Vital Signs and SAMPLE History information is presented in a table.

Initial Assessment information is presented in a table.

Fill-in-the-blank questions are interspersed throughout the case for students to answer as they read.

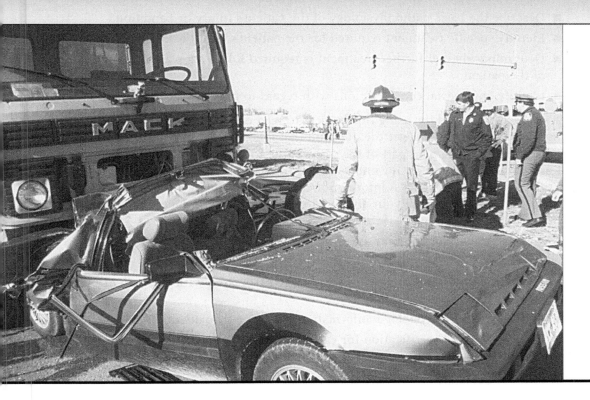

Introduction

Patient assessment and management combine to create an interwoven sequence of events that requires the paramedic to perform a systematic assessment of the patient and determine what treatment is most appropriate, and when it needs to be given.

Trauma Case Studies for the Paramedic contains 20 case studies representing a variety of trauma emergencies, some more life-threatening than others, that the paramedic may encounter in the field.

How to Use This book

Trauma Case Studies for the Paramedic is intended to reinforce the importance of a systematic patient assessment and management approach to paramedic students by presenting them with trauma emergencies that they are likely to encounter in the field. This book should be used as an additional resource for the paramedic student to test newly gained knowledge and prepare for examinations; it should not be used in place of a primary paramedic textbook.

Each case study will begin by presenting you with dispatch information, just as you would receive on an actual call, and a general impression of the patient upon arriving at the scene. Then, as the case progresses, pertinent patient information will be provided, interspersed with a series of questions designed to test your knowledge of the patient's specific injury or injuries. Students are asked to:

■ Describe the priorities of care based on the patient's clinical presentation.

■ Recognize the signs and symptoms of various injuries and conditions.

- Formulate a field impression based on the patient's signs and symptoms and findings of the rapid trauma assessment or focused history and physical examination.
- Describe the basic pathophysiology of the patient's injury or condition.
- Identify specific treatment required for the patient's injury or condition.
- Determine whether further treatment is required following reassessment of the patient.
- Identify any special considerations with regard to patient care or paramedic safety.

A suggested method for using this book is to read each part of the scenario, and then, in the area provided, answer the question that follows in as much detail as possible prior to reading the next part of the case study. Your detailed response to the questions will help reinforce your knowledge of the material. Continue this until you have read all of the scenario information and answered all of the case study questions. You should then compare your answers to those outlined in the case summary that immediately follows each case study.

The case summary provides answers to the questions asked within the case, as well as additional enrichment information, to include the following:

- Additional signs and symptoms commonly associated with the patient's injury or condition.
- Additional pathophysiologic information regarding the patient's injury or condition.
- Information and justification for each treatment modality.

Treatment Guidelines
The treatment recommendations contained within this book conform to the current standards of care as outlined in the following:

- US DOT EMT-Paramedic National Standard Curriculum, revised 1998
- American Heart Association Guidelines and Algorithms, revised 2000
- Brain Trauma Foundation (BTF), 2003

Additional treatment or variations in treatment may be required for each of the injuries presented in this book. As with the management of any patient, the paramedic must conform to the protocols inherent to his or her own EMS system, and should contact medical control as needed.

Body Substance Isolation (BSI) Precautions and Scene Safety
Strict adherence to proper body substance isolation (BSI) precautions and constantly observing the scene for safety hazards is of paramount importance when managing any patient. Throughout each of the case studies presented in this book, it is assumed that the proper BSI precautions are being followed at all times. Unless otherwise stated in the case study, it is also assumed that the scene is safe for you to enter.

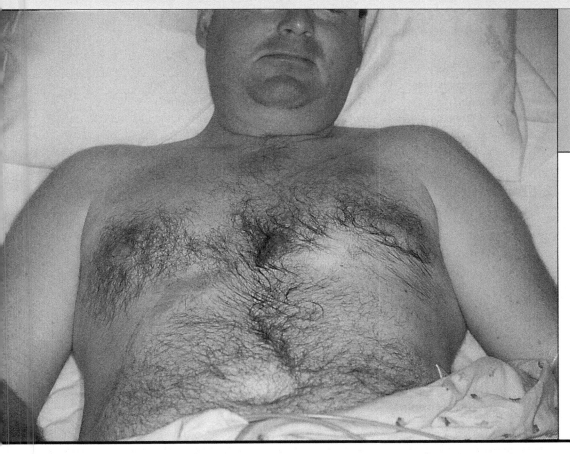

1

47-Year-Old Male Struck with a Steel Pipe

At 2:10 AM, you and your paramedic partner are dispatched to a local nightclub where an assault has occurred. Two law enforcement officers are at the scene, but they have not given you a situation update. Your response time to the scene is approximately 5 minutes.

1. What are your immediate concerns while responding to this call?

_____

_____

_____

_____

Your unit and two additional law enforcement officers arrive at the scene at the same time. You and your partner are escorted to the patient by the nightclub manager. You find a 47-year-old man who is conscious and alert and in moderate respiratory distress. The patient tells you that he was hit in the chest with a steel pipe. You note a large abrasion across his chest. Your partner obtains additional information from the manager as you perform an initial assessment **(Table 1-1)**.

Table 1-1 Initial Assessment

Mechanism of Injury	Blunt chest trauma
Level of Consciousness	Conscious and alert to person, place, and time
Chief Complaint	"My chest hurts, especially when I breathe."
Airway and Breathing	Airway is patent; respirations, increased and labored.
Circulation	Pulse is of normal rate, but irregular; skin, cool; no gross bleeding.

2. Based solely on the mechanism of injury, what injuries should you suspect?

_____

_____

_____

_____

You determine that the mechanism of injury warrants a rapid trauma assessment **(Table 1-2)**. Your partner places the patient on the cardiac monitor **(Figure 1-1)** and administers 100% supplemental oxygen with a nonrebreathing mask.

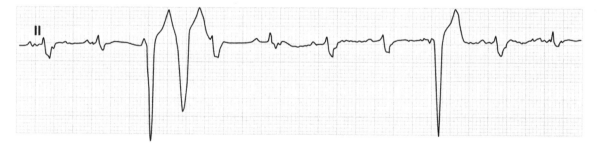

■ **Figure 1-1** Your patient's cardiac rhythm.

Table 1-2 Rapid Trauma Assessment

Head	No obvious trauma
Neck	Trachea is midline, jugular veins are normal, no cervical spine deformities.
Chest	Large abrasion over the precordial area; crepitus, bruising, and pain over the midsternum; breath sounds, clear and equal bilaterally to auscultation.
Abdomen/Pelvis	Abdomen is soft and nontender, pelvis is stable.
Lower Extremities	No obvious trauma, perfusion and sensory/motor function are grossly intact.
Upper Extremities	No obvious trauma, perfusion and sensory/motor function are grossly intact.
Posterior	No obvious trauma

The patient continues to complain of severe chest pain, especially when taking a breath. Although he remains conscious, you note that his respirations have become shallow and the pulse oximeter reads 85%, despite supplemental oxygen therapy.

3. How should you treat this patient's shallow breathing and low oxygen saturation?

_____

_____

_____

_____

Following your intervention, the patient's oxygen saturation has increased to 95%. Although restless, he remains conscious and is compliant with your intervention.

Your partner obtains baseline vital signs and a SAMPLE history **(Table 1-3)** and reports the findings to you.

Table 1-3 Baseline Vital Signs and SAMPLE History

Blood Pressure	134/74 mm Hg
Pulse	94 beats/min, strong and irregular
Respirations	24 breaths/min, labored and shallow (baseline); ventilations are being assisted.
Oxygen Saturation	95% (ventilated with 100% oxygen)
Signs and Symptoms	Chest pain, shortness of breath, blunt chest trauma
Allergies	No allergies
Medications	Topral
Pertinent Past History	Back surgery 2 years ago, hypertension
Last Oral Intake	"I had supper 2 hours ago."
Events Leading to the Injury	"I was attacked by two men as I was leaving the nightclub. They stole my wallet and then hit me in the chest with a steel pipe."

4. What is your field impression of this patient?

_____

_____

_____

_____

_____

5. What is the basis for your field impression?

_____

_____

_____

The patient is placed onto the stretcher and loaded into the ambulance. You begin transport to a hospital that is located 20 miles away. En route, you start an IV of normal saline and set the flow rate to keep the vein open.

6. What additional treatment should you provide for this patient?

_____

_____

_____

The patient's condition improves somewhat during transport. After administering additional care, you perform a detailed physical examination **(Table 1-4)**. The patient's breathing depth has improved, so you continue 100% oxygen with a nonrebreathing mask.

Table 1-4 Detailed Physical Examination

Head and Face	No obvious trauma to the scalp; ears, nose, and mouth are clear; pupils are midpoint, equal, and reactive to light.
Neck	Trachea is midline, jugular veins are normal, no cervical spine deformities.
Chest	Large abrasion over the precordial area; crepitus, bruising, and pain over the midsternum; breath sounds, clear and equal bilaterally to auscultation.
Abdomen/Pelvis	Abdomen is soft and nontender, pelvis is stable.
Lower Extremities	No obvious trauma, perfusion and sensory/motor function are grossly intact.
Upper Extremities	No obvious trauma, perfusion and sensory/motor function are grossly intact.
Posterior	No obvious trauma

You continue to monitor the patient's cardiac rhythm as well as the other interventions you have performed. After performing an ongoing assessment **(Table 1-5)**, you call your radio report to the receiving facility.

Table 1-5 Ongoing Assessment

Level of Consciousness	Conscious and alert to person, place, and time
Airway and Breathing	Airway remains patent; respirations, 22 breaths/min and slightly labored.
Oxygen Saturation	96% (on 100% oxygen)
Blood Pressure	130/70 mm Hg
Pulse	80 beats/min, strong and occasionally irregular
ECG	Sinus rhythm with occasional uniformed PVCs

The patient is delivered to the emergency department in stable condition. You give your verbal report to the attending physician, who orders a 12-lead ECG and a chest radiograph. The patient is diagnosed with a partial sternal fracture and a myocardial contusion. After being observed in the telemetry unit for 2 days, he is admitted to a regular room and then discharged home the next day.

CASE STUDY ANSWERS AND SUMMARY

1. What are your immediate concerns while responding to this call?

Your first and foremost concern, of course, is the safety of you and your partner. Although law enforcement is already at the scene, they have provided you with no information regarding the extent of injuries, the number of patients, or whether the scene is even secure. You must never assume that law enforcement presence ensures a safe scene, especially when the scene is a site for mass gatherings (eg, nightclubs, sporting events). You may inadvertently walk right into the middle of a group of hostile nightclub patrons! It would be prudent to wait until you receive a situation report from the on-scene police officers prior to entering the scene. If they don't immediately offer information about the scene, ask.

2. Based solely on the mechanism of injury, what injuries should you suspect?

Among others, blunt trauma to the chest could result in the following, potentially life-threatening, injuries:

- Flail chest
- Pneumothorax
- Pericardial tamponade
- Myocardial or pulmonary contusion
- Traumatic dissection of the thoracic aorta

Maintaining a high index of suspicion and performing a careful systematic assessment are critical aspects of management for the patient with blunt chest trauma. You must be prepared to treat all life-threatening injuries immediately upon discovery.

3. How should you treat this patient's shallow breathing and low oxygen saturation?

This patient is showing signs of inadequate breathing, as evidenced by the shallow depth of his respirations and his low oxygen saturation (SpO_2) level of 85%. At this point, you should assist his breathing attempts with a bag-valve-mask device attached to 100% oxygen. Advise the patient that each time he inhales, you will squeeze the bag-valve-mask device to increase the depth of his respirations. Continue assisted ventilations as necessary to maintain adequate tidal volume and an oxygen saturation of at least 90%.

Musculoskeletal trauma to the chest can make breathing a very difficult task for the patient. In fact, the pain with breathing may be so severe that the patient may voluntarily breathe with shallow depth (reduced tidal volume) in an attempt to minimize the pain. Prolonged shallow breathing may result in hypoxia and will require some form of positive-pressure ventilatory assistance, which is most effectively performed with a bag-valve-mask device. Because of the risk of barotrauma, you should avoid the use of any oxygen-powered ventilatory devices (eg, a demand valve).

4. What is your field impression of this patient?

On the basis of the mechanism of injury and the patient's clinical presentation, you should suspect the following injuries:

- Fractured sternum
- Myocardial contusion

5. What is the basis for your field impression?

The mechanism of injury, as with any type of trauma, should serve as your primary source when determining what injuries you suspect the patient may have. In the case of this particular patient, several key findings support a field impression of a sternal fracture and myocardial contusion:

- **Crepitus, bruising, and pain over the sternum.** These are all reliable indicators of an underlying sternal fracture.
  - It takes significant force to fracture the sternum, so one could easily see how the myocardium could have been injured.

- **Premature ventricular complexes (PVCs).** This patient is displaying a sinus rhythm with three PVCs, two of which occur in a row (couplet). PVCs associated with a myocardial contusion could indicate myocardial injury and irritability and should be looked at as a warning sign of a potentially life-threatening dysrhythmia, such as ventricular tachycardia or ventricular fibrillation.
  - Myocardial contusions are commonly associated with tachycardia. This patient, however, is taking topral (Metoprolol) for his hypertension. Topral is a beta adrenergic antagonist (beta blocker) that suppresses the sympathetic nervous system and blocks the release of epinephrine (adrenalin) and norepinephrine. This would explain the absence of tachycardia in this patient.

Myocardial contusions are commonly associated with blunt chest trauma, yet because of other, more obvious injuries, they are frequently overlooked.

A common mechanism of injury that causes contusions of the myocardium is a motor vehicle crash, when the chest strikes a fixed object, such as the steering wheel, or when an object strikes the chest, such as a baseball bat or steel pipe. Multiple rib fractures and sternal fractures are occasionally associated with myocardial contusion.

The severity of the injury may range from a localized contusion that produces no signs or symptoms to extensive myocardial injury associated with bleeding and edema, which could cause myocardial rupture. Bleeding may also occur into the pericardial sac, resulting in a pericardial tamponade.

If the patient is symptomatic, the signs and symptoms will typically be similar to those of an acute myocardial infarction (AMI) and can vary in severity **(Table 1-6)**. Of most concern to the paramedic should be the risk of lethal cardiac dysrhythmias. Areas in and around the contused myocardium become ischemic and can serve as the focal point for a variety of cardiac dysrhythmias, the most serious being ventricular tachycardia and ventricular fibrillation. If the area of contusion is large, myocardial contractility, stroke volume, and cardiac output can become significantly impaired, leading to cardiogenic shock.

Table 1-6 Signs and Symptoms of Myocardial Contusion

Bruising or abrasions over the precordium
Chest pain, pressure, or discomfort (similar to an AMI)
Tachycardia and palpitations
Diaphoresis
Hypotension (severe cases)
Ventricular dysrhythmias (severe cases)
Cardiogenic shock (rare)

Emergency care for the patient with a myocardial contusion is similar to that of the patient with an acute myocardial infarction and includes 100% oxygen, continuous cardiac monitoring (12-lead ECG if possible), and prompt transport. Should cardiac arrest develop, electrical and pharmacological therapy (eg, defibrillation, epinephrine) should be initiated. Follow standard advanced cardiac life support (ACLS) protocols and contact medical control as needed.

Because of the potential severity of the injury, any actions that increase myocardial oxygen demand and consumption, such as patient agitation, should be avoided.

6. What additional treatment should you provide for this patient?

- **Intravenous line of normal saline**
  - Because the patient's blood pressure is stable (134/74 mm Hg), fluid boluses are not required at this point. Set the flow rate of the IV to keep the vein open and monitor the patient for hypotension.
  - Intravenous access is necessary should the patient develop life-threatening cardiac dysrhythmias that would require pharmacological treatment with antidysrhythmics such as lidocaine or amiodarone.
- **Ventilatory support as needed**
  - If the patient continues to have shallow breathing due to the pain associated with the injury, continued positive-pressure ventilatory assistance will be necessary. Closely monitor the patient's breathing rate and depth and oxygen saturation.
  - Should the patient develop severe hypoxia and become unconscious, endotracheal intubation may be required to protect his airway from aspiration.
- **Continuous cardiac monitoring**
  - The PVCs that the patient is currently experiencing may indicate an impending lethal cardiac dysrhythmia, such as ventricular tachycardia or ventricular fibrillation. You must be prepared to perform defibrillation or cardioversion, if needed.
  - A 12-lead ECG should be obtained and assessed for ST-segment elevation/depression and T-wave inversion. Such changes indicate myocardial ischemia and injury.
- **Lidocaine**
  - Because this patient has evidence of myocardial irritability (eg, coupled PVCs) with signs of a myocardial contusion, you should administer lidocaine.
  - Begin with a bolus dose of 1 to 1.5 mg/kg IV push, followed by a lidocaine infusion of 1 to 4 mg/min. If ventricular irritability persists or worsens, consider additional boluses at 0.5 to 0.75 mg/kg IV push, and then titrate the infusion accordingly.

Summary

In contrast to penetrating trauma, where the injuries are obvious, blunt chest trauma is more commonly fatal. This is because it often presents with minimal or no external signs of injury. It is of utmost importance that the paramedic consider the mechanism of injury and perform a careful and systematic assessment of the patient with blunt chest trauma.

Vital anatomical structures that are commonly injured in the thoracic cavity include the heart, lungs, trachea, great vessels, and, in the lower aspect of the thoracic cavity, the liver. Any of these structures can be injured following blunt trauma to the chest.

The goals of managing a patient with a myocardial contusion include maintaining effective oxygenation and ventilation, monitoring for cardiac dysrhythmias, and promptly transporting the patient to the hospital. The presence of PVCs following a myocardial contusion indicates ventricular irritability and should be treated with lidocaine to prevent more lethal dysrhythmias (eg, V-Fib, V-Tach). Cautious use of intravenous fluid boluses is recommended. Unnecessarily increasing the patient's blood pressure can exacerbate intrathoracic bleeding, if present.

If the patient develops cardiac arrest, follow standard basic and advanced cardiac life support guidelines, including CPR and intubation, epinephrine, antidysrhythmics, and defibrillation.

2

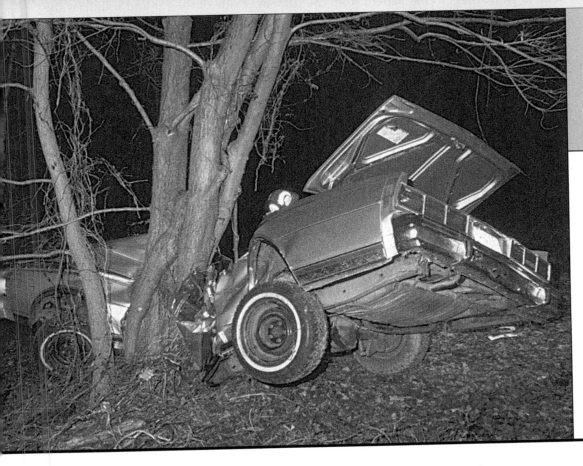

30-Year-Old Male with Severe Head Trauma

At 11:45 PM, your unit is dispatched to County Road 309 for a motor-vehicle accident. Law enforcement is at the scene; they advise you that there is one patient who is trapped in the car. He is breathing and has a pulse; however, his mental status is altered. Your response time to the scene is approximately 12 minutes.

1. **Based on the information from law enforcement, what additional resources should you request? Why?**

_____

_____

_____

_____

After arriving at the scene and surveying for any hazards, you approach the vehicle, which evidently slid off the road and struck a tree on the driver's side. Your partner is able to gain access to the patient from the passenger side of the car and stabilizes the patient's head. Rescue units arrive while you are performing an initial assessment of the patient (Table 2-1).

Table 2-1 Initial Assessment

Mechanism of Injury	Motor-vehicle crash with entrapment
Level of Consciousness	Responsive to painful stimuli only
Chief Complaint	Decreased level of consciousness, possible trauma to multiple body systems
Airway and Breathing	Airway is maintained by your partner, blood is flowing from the mouth, respirations are rapid and irregular.
Circulation	Pulse is slow and bounding, skin is warm and moist, bleeding is noted from the mouth and nose and from a large laceration to the left side of the head.

You immediately suction the patient's oropharynx and administer 100% oxygen with a nonrebreathing mask. A trauma dressing is placed on the left side of the patient's head to control the bleeding and a cervical collar is applied. Once freed from the wreckage, the patient is rapidly extricated from the car on a long spine board and placed on the ground.

2. What immediate management should be performed as soon as the patient is removed from the vehicle?

_____

_____

_____

_____

Your partner manages the patient's airway while you perform a rapid trauma assessment (Table 2-2). A firefighter advises you that the Med-Evac helicopter will be at the scene in approximately 5 minutes.

Table 2-2 Rapid Trauma Assessment

Head	Laceration (bleeding controlled) and depression to left side of the head, blood flowing from the mouth and nose, pupils are 4 mm and bilaterally sluggish in reaction to light.
Neck	Trachea is midline; jugular veins are normal, no cervical spine deformities.
Chest	Chest wall is stable to palpation, abrasions to left anterolateral chest, breath sounds are clear and equal bilaterally to auscultation.
Abdomen/Pelvis	Abdomen is soft and nontender, pelvis is stable.
Lower Extremities	Closed deformity to left midshaft femur; pedal pulses, bilaterally present
Upper Extremities	Multiple abrasions to the left lateral upper arm; radial pulses, bilaterally present
Posterior	No obvious trauma

After completing the rapid trauma assessment, the patient's spine is fully immobilized and he is placed into the ambulance. Because he has a Glasgow Coma Score of 8 **(Table 2-3)**, you and your partner agree that the patient needs to be intubated. While your partner is preparing the intubation equipment, you apply a cardiac monitor and assess the patient's ECG rhythm **(Figure 2-1)**. Next, you obtain a set of baseline vital signs and gather as much information as you can for a SAMPLE history **(Table 2-4)**.

Table 2-3 Your Patient's Glasgow Coma Score

Eye opening	Responds to pain (2)
Verbal response	Incomprehensible sounds (2)
Motor response	Withdraws from pain (4)

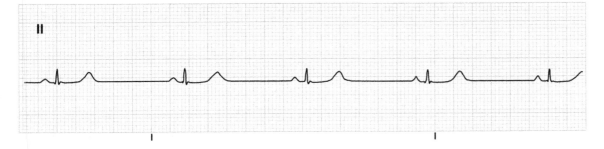

■ **Figure 2-1** Your patient's cardiac rhythm.

Table 2-4 Baseline Vital Signs and SAMPLE History

Blood Pressure	190/104 mm Hg
Pulse	44 beats/min, regular and bounding
Respirations	30 breaths/min and irregular (baseline), ventilated with 100% oxygen
Oxygen Saturation	96% (ventilated with 100% oxygen)
Signs and Symptoms	Decreased mental status, inadequate breathing, laceration and depression to the skull, bradycardia, and hypertension
Allergies	The patient is wearing a medic alert bracelet stating that he is allergic to penicillin.
Medications	Unknown
Pertinent Past History	Unknown
Last Oral Intake	Unknown
Events Leading to the Injury	Unknown. There were no witnesses to the event.

3. Why is nasotracheal intubation contraindicated in this patient?

4. Should this patient be hyperventilated? Why or why not?

The patient has been successfully intubated and is being ventilated at the appropriate rate by your partner. You can hear the approaching aircraft as you initiate an IV line of normal saline with a 16-gauge IV catheter.

5. What is appropriate with regard to intravenous fluid management for this patient?

_____

_____

_____

_____

Shortly after securing the IV line, one of the flight paramedics opens the back door of the ambulance. After briefing the flight paramedic on the patient's condition, he asks you to accompany him with the patient for assistance. You move the patient to the awaiting helicopter, where he is immediately transported to a trauma center that is 40 miles away.

6. What is the pathophysiology of this patient's injury?

_____

_____

_____

_____

En route to the hospital, the flight paramedic places the patient on an automatic transport ventilator (ATV) and sets the ventilatory rate while you obtain a repeat blood pressure, which is 170/94 mm Hg. The patient's pulse rate is 70 beats per minute, and his oxygen saturation is 97%.

Upon arriving at the trauma center, you are met by an emergency department physician and a trauma surgeon. After further stabilization in the emergency department, a computer tomographic (CT) scan of the head reveals a depressed fracture of the left temporal skull and an epidural hemorrhage. Following surgical intervention to control bleeding from the damaged artery, the patient is admitted to the surgical intensive care unit. Following extensive rehabilitative care, the patient recovered with only a mild neurological deficit.

CASE STUDY ANSWERS AND SUMMARY

1. Based on the information from law enforcement, what additional resources should you request? Why?

With a response time of 12 minutes and a patient who is entrapped in his vehicle, rescue personnel able to extricate the patient from the vehicle should also be dispatched to the scene. According to the law enforcement officer's information, this situation may require specialized rescue equipment and appropriately trained personnel. Because extrication of this patient may be lengthy and his mental status is already altered, you should consider requesting aeromedical evacuation, which can save valuable time in getting the patient to a trauma center. You should thoroughly understand your local protocols for requesting this type of support. In most circumstances, they will be dispatched automatically for this type of call, and requests for additional resources will be made through the incident commander on the scene or the senior responding paramedic.

2. What immediate management should be performed as soon as the patient is removed from the vehicle?

Recall from the initial assessment that this patient had blood in his oropharynx and inadequate breathing (eg, rapid and irregular breaths). As soon as the patient is removed from the vehicle, your partner should, while maintaining in-line stabilization of the patient's head with his knees, resuction the oropharynx and begin assisting ventilations with a bag-valve-mask (BVM) device and 100% oxygen. Because the patient is unconscious, an airway adjunct should be inserted to further maintain airway patency. Endotracheal intubation should also be considered, but not before the airway has been managed utilizing basic means (eg, BVM ventilation).

If the oral secretions are continuous, your partner should suction the patient's oropharynx for 15 seconds and then assist ventilations for 2 minutes. This alternating pattern should continue until the secretions are cleared from the airway or the patient is intubated. It is imperative that the patient's airway remain patent at all times.

3. Why is nasotracheal intubation contraindicated in this patient?

This patient likely has a skull fracture and is bleeding from the nose, both of which are contraindications to nasotracheal intubation. Blood draining from the nose following head trauma could contain cerebrospinal fluid (cerebrospinal rhinorrhea), which would indicate a fracture of the cribriform plate. The cribriform plate forms a portion of the base of the cranium. Any tube inserted nasally could inadvertently enter the cranium through the fractured cribriform plate, thus causing direct damage to the brain. Both nasotracheal intubation and nasogastric tube insertion are contraindicated in patients with midface fractures, cerebrospinal fluid drainage from the nose, and possible cribriform plate injuries.

Other signs of a skull fracture, which are typically later manifestations, include periorbital ecchymosis **(Figure 2-2)**, also referred to as "raccoon's eyes," and retroauricular ecchymosis **(Figure 2-3)**, also referred to as "Battle's sign." These signs often take several hours to develop after a skull fracture; their absence should not be taken as an indication that a skull fracture is not present.

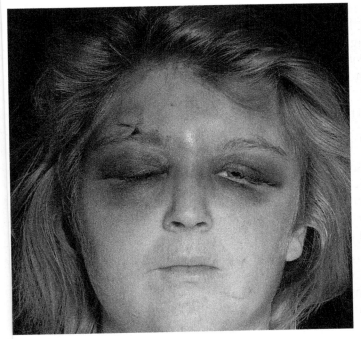

■ **Figure 2-2** Periorbital ecchymosis (raccoon's eyes).

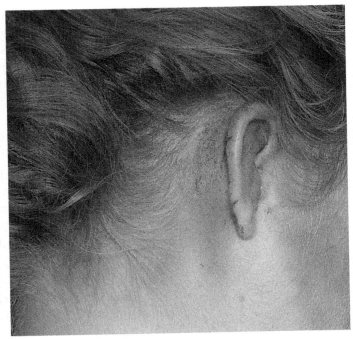

■ **Figure 2-3** Retroauricular ecchymosis (Battle's sign).

4. Should this patient be hyperventilated? Why or why not?

The goal of airway management for the brain-injured patient with increased intracranial pressure (ICP) is first and foremost to maintain oxygenation and ventilation, and second, to maintain cerebral perfusion pressure (CPP). Unless the patient is exhibiting signs of brain herniation **(Table 2-5)**, ventilations should occur at a rate of 10 breaths per minute while maintaining an oxygen saturation (SpO$_2$) of greater than 90%. According to the Brain Trauma Foundation (BTF), a *single* drop in the patient's SpO$_2$ below 90% doubles the adult brain-injured patient's chance of death.

Hyperventilating the patient would cause decreased blood levels of carbon dioxide (PaCO$_2$), resulting in cerebral vasoconstriction. Although this may decrease ICP, it also has the effect of decreasing cerebral blood flow, and may therefore potentially decrease overall cerebral perfusion. In patients with markedly elevated intracranial pressure and signs of impending herniation, hyperventilation for short periods of time may be effective.

Table 2-5 Signs of Brain Herniation

Unresponsive (comatose) patient, with
- Bilateral unresponsive (fixed) pupils **or** asymmetric pupils, **AND** any one of the following:
  - Abnormal extension (decerebrate posturing)
  - No motor response to painful stimuli (flaccid paralysis)
  - Hemiplegia (paralysis to one half of the body)

Hypertension and bradycardia are often present.

If signs of brain herniation are present, the adult patient should be hyperventilated at a rate of 20 breaths per minute. Clearly, this is a last ditch attempt to cause a rapid decrease in ICP (at the expense of CPP), thus buying some time until neurosurgical intervention.

5. What is appropriate with regard to intravenous fluid management for this patient?

This patient's vital signs (eg, hypertension, bradycardia) indicate the body's compensatory response to significant ICP; therefore, intravenous fluids should be restricted *at this particular point in time*. In the absence of hypotension, intravenous fluids should be restricted in the head-injured patient in order to minimize cerebral edema and ICP.

Hypotension (SBP <90 mm Hg), however, if present in the patient with increased ICP, can significantly reduce CPP, and should be managed with crystalloid fluid boluses of 20 mL/kg to maintain a systolic blood pressure of at least 90 mm Hg.

The critical minimum threshold for CPP is 60 mm Hg, which means that anything less is associated with brain-cell death. CPP is computed by subtracting the patient's ICP, the upper limit of normal being 15 mm Hg, from the mean arterial pressure (MAP). MAP is calculated using the following formula:

$$\text{MAP} = \text{Systolic blood pressure} + (2 \times \text{Diastolic blood pressure})$$

Although ICP cannot be measured in the field, let's assume that in this particular patient it is 20 mm Hg (it should be no greater than 15 mm Hg). To demonstrate the deleterious effects of hypotension, we will calculate his CPP, using both his last blood pressure reading of 170/94 mm Hg and a hypotensive blood pressure of 90/50 mm Hg. Bear in mind that a CPP of less than 60 mm Hg is associated with brain-cell death:

- **CPP based on a blood pressure of 170/94 mm Hg:**
  - 170 (SBP) + 2 × 94 (DBP) = 358 ÷ 3 = MAP of 119
  - 119 (MAP) − 20 mm Hg (ICP) = **CPP of 99**
- **CPP based on a blood pressure of 90/50 mm Hg:**
  - 90 (SBP) + 2 × 50 (DBP) = 190 ÷ 3 = MAP of 63
  - 63 (MAP) − 20 mm Hg (ICP) = **CPP of 43**

From these examples, it is clear that hypotension in the brain-injured patient could be lethal and therefore must be aggressively managed. In fact, according to the BTF, a *single* drop in systolic blood pressure to less than 90 mm Hg doubles the adult brain-injured patient's chance of death.

Dextrose-containing solutions, such as 5% dextrose in water (D_5W), should not be administered to a patient with a traumatic brain injury. D_5W is a hypertonic solution, which would draw fluid from the cells and into the vascular space, thus exacerbating cerebral edema and ICP.

The ultimate goal of intravenous therapy in the head-injured patient is to maintain CPP without exacerbating ICP. Because this can be a fine balance to maintain, your intravenous line(s) must be titrated carefully and you must constantly monitor the patient.

6. What is the pathophysiology of this patient's injury?

This patient appears to be suffering from an epidural hemorrhage. This type of injury is the result of bleeding between the dura mater and the interior surface of the skull **(Figure 2-4)** and often involves a tear of the middle meningeal artery in the temporal region. Epidural hematomas are commonly associated with depressed skull fractures of the temporal bone.

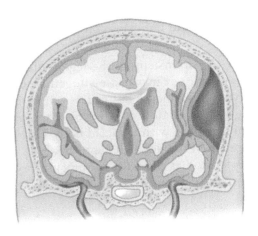

■ **Figure 2-4**
Epidural hematoma.

Because the origin of the bleeding is an artery, ICP builds and rapidly compresses the cerebrum and other associated structures (eg, the brainstem). As ICP increases further, the body's ability to maintain CPP is compromised, and cerebral blood flow is diminished.

Through a process called autoregulation, the body attempts to compensate for the fall in CPP by increasing systemic blood pressure and dilating the cerebral vasculature, thus shunting more blood to the brain. However, this increase in cerebral blood flow further increases ICP. Eventually, the body's compensatory mechanisms will fail, and the blood pressure (and CPP) will begin to fall.

If left untreated, ICP may cause the brain to herniate. Herniation can occur over the tentorium (one of the three extensions of the dura mater that separates the cerebellum from the occipital lobe of the cerebrum) or through the foramen magnum (the large opening at the base of the skull).

The signs of increasing ICP depend on the area of the brainstem involved **(Table 2-6)**. Early signs of increased ICP include headache, nausea and vomiting, and alterations in mentation. As ICP increases further, the patient develops hypertension, bradycardia, and abnormal respiratory patterns (Cushing's triad). Compression of the hypothalamus may result in vomiting (often without nausea) and fluctuations in body temperature.

Posturing indicates brainstem compression and presents as either flexion of the arms and extension of the legs (decorticate posturing) or extension of both the arms and legs (decerebrate posturing). Compression of the brainstem also produces abnormal respiratory patterns. Cheyne-Stokes respirations are characterized by periods of rapid and slow breathing with alternating periods of apnea **(Figure 2-5)**. Cheyne-Stokes respirations often accompany decorticate posturing and are indicative of upper brainstem compression.

Cheyne-Stokes breathing

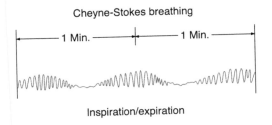

Inspiration/expiration

■ **Figure 2-5** Cheyne-Stokes respirations in a head-injured patient indicate possible upper brainstem compression.

Central neurogenic hyperventilation, which is characterized by deep, rapid breathing, may accompany decerebrate posturing and indicates compression of the middle portion of the brainstem.

When pressure is placed on the lower brainstem, in the region of the medulla oblongata, respirations become erratic (ataxic) or may cease altogether. Compression and paralysis of the oculomotor nerve (cranial nerve III) causes one or both pupils to become fixed (nonreactive to light) and dilated. At this point, the patient is completely unconscious and unresponsive with a flaccid body. Other findings associated with lower brainstem compression include ECG abnormalities (eg, QRS, ST-segment, T-wave changes) and hypotension as the body's compensatory mechanisms to maintain CPP fail. Obviously, most patients do not survive this level of intracranial pressure.

Table 2-6 Signs of Increased Intracranial Pressure

Upper brainstem compression
- Hypertension and bradycardia
- Pupils typically remain reactive
- Cheyne-Stokes respirations
- Withdrawal from pain with decorticate posturing
- Good prognosis with prompt intervention

Middle brainstem compression
- Widened pulse pressure and bradycardia
- Sluggish or nonreactive pupils
- Central neurogenic hyperventilation
- Decerebrate posturing
- Patient typically suffers permanent neurologic deficit, even with prompt intervention.

Lower brainstem compression
- Fixed and dilated pupils (on one or both sides)
- Ataxic (erratic) respirations
- Patient is unconscious, unresponsive, and flaccid.
- ECG abnormalities
- Hypotension
- Typically a fatal event

Summary

The cranium is a rigid, unyielding box that protects the brain from minor head injuries. The brain occupies approximately 80% of the intracranial space. When intracranial bleeding occurs, such as that seen with an epidural hemorrhage, that same unyielding box does not expand; therefore, the brain and its vital structures are compressed, and CPP is compromised.

In contrast to diffuse brain injury, in which movement of the brain within the skull secondary to acceleration or deceleration forces causes injury to the brain and its motor nerve cells (axonal injury), injuries such as an epidural hematoma would be classified as a focal injury and are typically the result of direct impact to a localized part of the skull, such as the patient in this case study, whose head most likely struck the B-post of the car when it broadsided the tree. However, if bleeding from an intracranial hemorrhage is severe, the entire brain, including its vital structures, will be compressed by ICP.

The adult patient's cranium can accommodate a relatively small amount of blood. After a certain degree of ICP occurs due to bleeding, the patient's condition deteriorates. If not treated promptly, ICP will force the brain through an opening (herniation), and the patient will die.

General treatment guidelines for the head-injured patient include ensuring a patent airway with simultaneous spinal protection and maintaining adequate oxygenation and ventilation. Provide positive-pressure ventilations at a rate of 10 breaths per minute to the inadequately breathing patient, but remember, do not hyperventilate unless signs of herniation are present. Intubate the patient if his Glasgow Coma Scale is less than 8, he is unconscious, or his airway is otherwise compromised. If the patient is breathing adequately (good rate and tidal volume), 100% supplemental oxygen with a nonrebreathing mask should be administered. Whether you are ventilating the patient or administering passive oxygen with a nonrebreathing mask, maintain the patient's oxygen saturation at 90% or greater.

Unless the head-injured patient is hypotensive (SBP <90 mm Hg), intravenous fluids should be restricted, because excessive fluids may exacerbate ICP. If hypotension exists, isotonic crystalloids should be infused at a rate of 20 mL/kg to maintain a systolic blood pressure of at least 90 mm Hg. Dextrose-containing solutions, such as 5% dextrose in water (D_5W), should not be administered to the patient with head injury and intracranial pressure.

Other management for the head-injured patient includes monitoring for hyperthermia and limiting external stimulation (eg, lights and siren). Agitation of the patient may further increase ICP or propagate a seizure. If seizures occur, administer a benzodiazepine (eg, Ativan, Valium). Monitor the patient's cardiac rhythm and be prepared to treat arrhythmias.

It cannot be overemphasized that rapid identification of a brain injury, prompt care in the field, and rapid transport to a trauma center for neurosurgical intervention are vital components in the successful management of the patient with severe head injury.

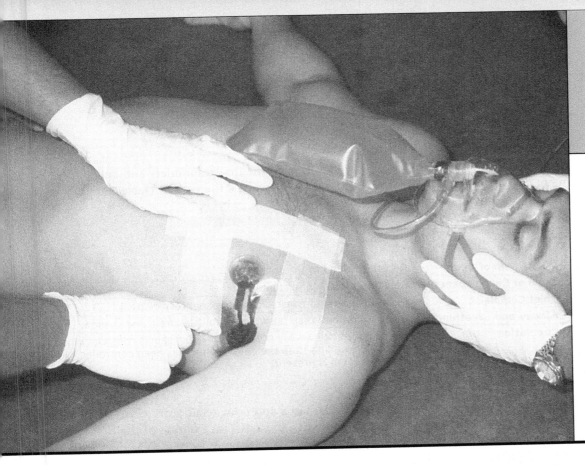

3

22-Year-Old Male with a Gunshot Wound to the Chest

At 10:50 AM, your unit is dispatched to a convenience store in response to a shooting. The shooting evidently occurred during a robbery attempt in which the clerk shot the perpetrator. Law enforcement is at the scene and notifies you by radio that the scene is secure and that first responders from the fire department are caring for the patient. Your response time to the scene is approximately 7 minutes.

You arrive at the scene at 10:57 AM, where you find the patient, a 22-year-old male who is semiconscious and in obvious respiratory distress. The patient is being cared for by first responders. They have already sealed a small caliber gunshot wound to the left side of his chest and placed him on 100% supplemental oxygen via a nonrebreathing mask. Because the patient reportedly fell to the ground after being shot, one of the first responders is maintaining manual stabilization of the patient's head.

1. Why is it important to immediately seal an open wound to the thoracic cavity?

_____

_____

_____

_____

Your partner gathers additional information from the first responders and law enforcement officers while you perform an initial assessment of the patient **(Table 3-1)**.

Table 3-1 Initial Assessment

Mechanism of Injury	Gunshot wound to the chest
Level of Consciousness	Responsive to painful stimuli only
Chief Complaint	Decreased level of consciousness, respiratory distress
Airway and Breathing	Airway is patent; respirations are rapid, labored, and shallow.
Circulation	Radial pulses are weakly present and rapid; skin is cool, clammy, and pale; bleeding from the chest wound has been controlled. No other bleeding is present.

Because of the patient's decreased mental status and poor respiratory effort, your partner inserts a nasopharyngeal airway and, with the assistance of one of the first responders, initiates positive-pressure ventilatory assistance with a BVM device and 100% oxygen.

2. What are the hazards of ventilating a chest-injury patient with a manually triggered ventilation device?

_____

_____

_____

_____

The patient's oxygen saturation reads 92% with assisted ventilation and 100% oxygen. While your partner continues positive-pressure ventilatory assistance, you perform a rapid trauma assessment to detect other potentially life-threatening injuries **(Table 3-2)**.

Table 3-2 Rapid Trauma Assessment

Head	No obvious trauma
Neck	Trachea is midline; jugular veins appear normal, no cervical spine deformities.
Chest	Open wound to the upper-left anterior chest (sealed); chest wall movement is asymmetrical; breath sounds are diminished over the upper-left anterior chest.
Abdomen/Pelvis	Abdomen is soft and nontender, pelvis is stable.
Lower Extremities	No obvious trauma, perfusion and sensory/motor function are grossly intact.
Upper Extremities	No obvious trauma, perfusion and sensory/motor function are grossly intact.
Posterior	No obvious trauma

After applying a cervical collar and fully immobilizing the patient with a long spine board, you quickly load him into the ambulance. While your partner obtains baseline vital signs and a SAMPLE history **(Table 3-3)**, you apply the ECG leads and assess the patient's cardiac rhythm **(Figure 3-1)**. Transport is begun to a trauma center that is 10 miles away. A first responder accompanies you in the back of the ambulance to assist with patient care. Because the injury occurred during the commission of a crime, a police officer also accompanies you in the ambulance.

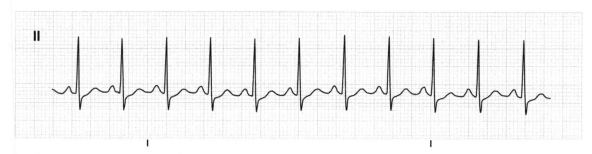

■ **Figure 3-1** Your patient's cardiac rhythm.

Table 3-3 Baseline Vital Signs and SAMPLE History

Blood Pressure	70/40 mm Hg
Pulse	128 beats/min, weak and regular
Respirations	28 breaths/min and shallow (ventilated with 100% oxygen)
Oxygen Saturation	89% (ventilated with 100% oxygen)
Signs and Symptoms	Open chest wound (sealed), signs of shock, inadequate breathing
Allergies	Unknown
Medications	Unknown
Pertinent Past History	Unknown
Last Oral Intake	Unknown
Events Leading to the Injury	According to the clerk, "He tried to rob me, so I shot him with my .22 caliber pistol that I keep behind the counter."

Because of the profound hypotension and decreasing oxygen saturation, you reauscultate the patient's breath sounds and note that they are absent on the entire left side. Additionally, you note that his jugular veins appear somewhat distended, his trachea has deviated to the right side, and his respirations have become increasingly labored. Because you are busy with patient care, you ask your partner, who is driving the ambulance, to notify the receiving facility of your impending arrival.

3. Why is this patient's condition deteriorating? What corrective action must you take?

You take immediate steps to correct the problem that is causing the patient's deterioration. Within minutes after your intervention, you note improvement in the patient's respiratory effort, and his oxygen saturation is now 94%. Additionally, his mental status has improved to the point where he will no longer tolerate assisted ventilation. You apply 100% oxygen via a nonrebreathing mask and are able to secure one large-bore IV line of normal saline. With a 5-minute estimated time of arrival at the trauma center, you perform a detailed physical examination **(Table 3-4)**.

Table 3-4 Detailed Physical Examination

Head and Face	No obvious trauma to the scalp; ears, nose, and mouth are clear; pupils are equal and reactive to light.
Neck	Trachea has now returned to the midline, jugular veins are less distended.
Chest	Chest wound is sealed, breath sounds are diminished in the upper-left anterior chest, and chest wall movement is slightly asymmetrical.
Abdomen/Pelvis	Abdomen is soft and nontender, pelvis is stable.
Lower Extremities	No obvious trauma, perfusion and sensory/motor function are grossly intact.
Upper Extremities	No obvious trauma, perfusion and sensory/motor function are grossly intact.
Posterior	Examined in the rapid trauma assessment. Patient is immobilized by long spine board.

The patient's condition remains stable. He is conscious and alert to person and place, but cannot remember what happened. After performing an ongoing assessment **(Table 3-5)**, you call your report to the emergency department, which is less than 1 minute away.

Table 3-5 Ongoing Assessment

Level of Consciousness	Conscious and alert to person and place, cannot remember preceding events
Airway and Breathing	Airway remains patent; respirations, 22 breaths/min and slightly labored
Oxygen Saturation	96% (on 100% oxygen)
Breath Sounds	Slightly diminished in upper-left anterior chest
Jugular Veins	Nondistended
Blood Pressure	118/66 mm Hg
Pulse	94 beats/min, strong and regular
ECG	Normal sinus rhythm

With law enforcement accompaniment, the patient is transferred to the care of the attending emergency department physician. Following additional assessment in the emergency department, a chest tube is placed, and the patient is admitted for treatment of his lung injury. After a 4-day stay in the hospital, the patient is discharged to the custody of law enforcement.

4. Describe the pathophysiology and emergency care of a tension pneumothorax.

_____

_____

_____

_____

1. Why is it important to immediately seal an open wound to the thoracic cavity?

Because of the mechanism of injury (gunshot wound to the chest) and the patient's obvious respiratory distress, you should suspect an open pneumothorax (sucking chest wound). An open pneumothorax develops when the pleural space is directly exposed to atmospheric pressure **(Figure 3-2)**.

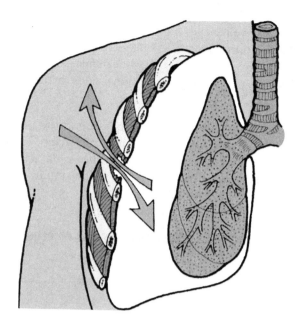

■ **Figure 3-2** A sucking chest wound allows air to enter the pleural space, thus preventing the lung from occupying the same space, impairing pulmonary gas exchange.

If the open chest wound is greater than or equal to two-thirds of the diameter of the opening between the vocal cords (glottic opening), atmospheric pressure will draw air through the chest wound and into the pleural space during inhalation (this is more common with high-caliber gunshot wounds). This will prevent air from entering the alveoli and participating in pulmonary gas exchange.

Immediate sealing of the wound with a nonporous (occlusive) dressing will prevent air from entering the pleural space, thus facilitating the entry of air into the lungs. The dressing should be secured on three sides, which will allow air to escape from the pleural space on exhalation but prevent air entry into the pleural space during inhalation.

It is important for the paramedic to remember that once a sucking chest wound is covered, it has been converted from an open pneumothorax to a closed one; therefore, close monitoring for signs of a developing tension pneumothorax is essential.

2. What are the hazards of ventilating a chest-injury patient with a manually triggered ventilation device?

Use of a manually triggered ventilation device, such as a flow-restricted oxygen-powered ventilation device (FROPVD), should be avoided when ventilating a patient with a chest injury. The FROPVD delivers oxygen under high pressure (40 liters per breath), which, by providing excessive tidal volume, could cause barotrauma and exacerbate the chest injury. A BVM device with a reservoir and supplemental oxygen is the preferred method for ventilating patients with chest trauma, regardless of whether the injury is open or closed.

3. Why is this patient's condition deteriorating? What corrective action must you take?

This patient's hemodynamic compromise is the result of a developing tension pneumothorax. The following signs and symptoms that the patient is experiencing confirms the presence of a tension pneumothorax:

- **Absent breath sounds on the ipsilateral (same) side of the injury**
  - This indicates that the entire lung has collapsed due to excessive pressure in the pleural space and is no longer capable of expanding during inhalation.

- **Hypotension**
  - When the pleural space fills with air and the affected lung collapses, pressure is exerted across the mediastinum to the opposite lung. During this process, both the myocardium and the aorta are compressed. As a result, stroke volume and cardiac output both fall and hypotension develops.

- **Jugular venous distention**
  - This is caused by impaired venous return to the right side of the heart (preload) due to compression of the vena cava. As a result, blood backs up beyond the right atrium, causing distention of the jugular veins.

- **Increased respiratory difficulty**
  - This is the result of the collapsed lungs' inability to expand. As a result, the patient is now attempting to breathe with only one functional lung. Oxygen saturation (SpO_2) is usually markedly low.

- **Asymmetrical chest wall movement**
  - Because one lung is collapsed, it will obviously not expand during inhalation. This causes the affected hemithorax (half of the chest) to remain stationary while the opposite hemithorax moves normally.

- **Tracheal deviation**
  - This is a classic sign of a tension pneumothorax, but unfortunately it occurs late. As the air between the pleural layers expands, the entire mediastinum and its contents are shifted to the side opposite the pneumothorax. As a result, the trachea follows, and tracheal deviation can be seen on exam.

As mentioned earlier, when sealing a sucking chest wound, you are converting an open pneumothorax to a closed one. As a result, pressure (tension) may continue to build within the pleural space, resulting in further collapse of the lung. *Immediate corrective action is to simply lift one side of the occlusive dressing to allow air to escape from the pleural space.* In most cases, this will improve the patient's condition. You may have to perform this procedure more than once during transport. If pleural tension is not released despite lifting the occlusive dressing, a needle thoracentesis, which will be discussed later in this case summary, will have to be performed.

4. Describe the pathophysiology and emergency care of a tension pneumothorax.

A tension pneumothorax is a life-threatening emergency that develops when air within the thoracic cavity cannot exit the pleural space. The result is severe respiratory distress, shock (hypoperfusion), and death if not recognized and immediately treated.

The visceral pleura lines the external lung tissue and the parietal pleura lines the thoracic cavity. Under normal circumstances, the visceral and parietal pleura are in contact with each other, with pleural fluid between each pleural layer facilitating frictionless movement. Because the pleura are in contact with one another, the space in between is a potential space, rather than an actual one.

Perforation of the lung, commonly from a fractured rib or a projectile such as a bullet, can occur during blunt or penetrating chest trauma. As a result, air exits the lung perforation and enters the space between the pleural layers during inhalation. On exhalation, the perforated lung acts as a one-way valve, thus preventing air from reentering the lung and exiting the pleural space. As pleural pressure increases, the lung progressively collapses, thus reducing pulmonary capacity—the amount of air that the lungs can hold **(Figure 3-3)**. As pulmonary capacity decreases, impairment of pulmonary gas exchange occurs, and the patient becomes increasingly dyspneic and hypoxic.

Once the injured lung has completely collapsed, tension is exerted laterally as well as across the mediastinum toward the opposite lung. During this process, the myocardium, aorta, and vena cava are compressed. Compression of these vital structures causes decreased venous return to the heart, decreased stroke volume (volume of blood ejected per ventricular contraction), and decreased cardiac output (volume of blood ejected from the heart each minute). As a result, the patient develops hypotension.

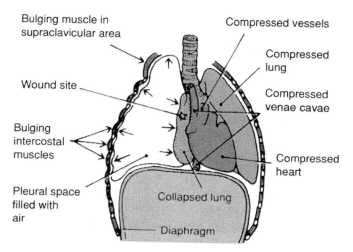

Bulging muscle in supraclavicular area

Compressed vessels

Wound site

Compressed lung

Compressed venae cavae

Bulging intercostal muscles

Compressed heart

Pleural space filled with air

Collapsed lung

Diaphragm

■ **Figure 3-3** During a tension pneumothorax, pulmonary capacity decreases as the lung collapses, impairing pulmonary gas exchange.

If tension is not immediately relieved from the pleural space, pressure will continue to increase and begin to affect the contralateral (opposite) lung, leading to its collapse as well. Shock (hypoperfusion) caused by a tension pneumothorax is "obstructive" in that it is caused by compression and obstruction of the myocardium and great vessels.

A tension pneumothorax can also develop following placement of an occlusive dressing over a sucking chest wound (open pneumothorax). Recall that sealing the wound converts it to a closed pneumothorax; tension can build within the pleural space. This is easily remedied by lifting a corner of the occlusive dressing to relieve pleural pressure. If lifting the dressing is unsuccessful, a needle thoracentesis will be required.

The signs and symptoms of a tension pneumothorax represent those of cardiovascular and respiratory system compromise **(Table 3-6)**. The paramedic must perform a careful, systematic assessment of the patient in order to recognize these signs and symptoms and provide immediate treatment.

Table 3-6 Signs and Symptoms of a Tension Pneumothorax

Increasing dyspnea and tachypnea
- Results from progressive collapsing of the lung and reduced lung capacity

Anxiety and restlessness
- Results from cerebral hypoxia

Cyanosis
- Caused by decreased oxygen levels in the arterial blood
- Cyanosis may not be present in the early stages of a tension pneumothorax.

Tachycardia
- Caused by a sympathetic nervous system release of epinephrine in an attempt to maintain adequate perfusion

Pallor and diaphoresis
- These are signs of shock, indicating discharge of the sympathetic nervous system, peripheral vasoconstriction and shunting of blood to vital organs, and activation of the sweat glands.

Hypotension
- Occurs as the result of decreased stroke volume and cardiac output
- Hypotension is typically not seen until the myocardium and great vessels have been compressed, which makes it a relatively later finding.

Diminished or absent breath sounds on the affected side
- A partially or completely collapsed lung does not have the ability to fully expand; therefore, tidal volume is markedly reduced.

Bulging intercostal muscles on the affected side
- This occurs as tension exerts laterally, but is inhibited by the ribs.

Jugular venous distention
- Caused by compression of the superior vena cava, with resultant decreased venous return to the right atrium
- Jugular venous distention is a later finding of a tension pneumothorax.

Asymmetrical chest wall movement
- The injured lung will not expand once it has completely collapsed; however, the unaffected lung continues to function normally. This produces uneven or asymmetrical expansion of the chest during inhalation.

Subcutaneous emphysema
- Because air cannot exit the pleural space, it is forced into the subcutaneous layers of the skin. This produces a crackling sensation upon palpation.

Tracheal deviation away from the affected side
- This is also a late finding in a tension pneumothorax. It occurs after the injured lung has completely collapsed and the air in the pleural cavity has pushed the mediastinum away from the side of the injury, pushing the trachea with it.
- You must not wait for tracheal deviation to occur before initiating treatment for a tension pneumothorax. It is typically a late sign.

Emergency care for a patient with a tension pneumothorax, which is summarized in **Table 3-7**, must be *immediate and aggressive*. Do not wait for later signs to develop, such as jugular venous distention, tracheal deviation, or hypotension, before initiating treatment.

Initial management includes ensuring a patent airway as well as adequate ventilation and oxygenation. If the patient is breathing adequately (eg, adequate rate and tidal volume), administer 100% supplemental oxygen via a nonrebreathing mask. If, however, the patient has poor respiratory effort, such as profound labored breathing or reduced tidal volume, positive-pressure ventilatory support must be initiated immediately. Intubation should be performed if the patient is unconscious. Continually monitor the patient's oxygen saturation.

Once adequate oxygenation and ventilation have been ensured, air from the pleural space must be evacuated as soon as possible. This involves performing a needle thoracentesis, also referred to as a chest decompression. Needle thoracentesis is accomplished by inserting a 2-inch, large-bore (12- or 14-gauge) IV catheter through the chest wall and into the affected pleural space. The proper insertion point is in between the second and third intercostal space, in the midclavicular line. The needle should be inserted above the third rib, because the inferior rib border is lined with intercostal vasculature and nerves. Following insertion of the needle, you should hear a rush of air as pressure is relieved from the pleural space, thus confirming the tension pneumothorax. You should also see marked improvement in the patient's condition, such as improved respiratory effort and oxygen saturation as the lung reexpands. Unless associated with internal bleeding, improvement in the patient's blood pressure will also be noted. If the tension is not relieved with the initial needle thoracentesis, insertion of a second or third needle may be warranted.

To ensure continued pleural evacuation and prevention of air reentry into the pleural space, attach a one-way valve to the hub of the intravenous catheter. This can be accomplished by a variety of methods, including the finger of a rubber glove or a commercially manufactured device.

Relative to other emergency care procedures, needle thoracentesis is an invasive technique; therefore, your medical director may require that you contact him or her prior to performing the procedure. Follow locally established protocols.

If air transport is utilized, you may often see the flight nurse or paramedic perform a needle thoracentesis in patients with a simple pneumothorax, even if they are hemodynamically stable. This is necessary because increased altitude will cause a simple pneumothorax to progress to a tension pneumothorax more rapidly than if the patient were transported by ground. Stable patients with a simple pneumothorax who are going to be ground transported typically will not require immediate needle thoracentesis.

Two large-bore (14- or 16-gauge) IV lines should be established; however, the shock associated with a tension pneumothorax is generally caused by obstruction of normal cardiopulmonary function, not hypovolemia. Needle thoracentesis has priority over intravenous therapy for the unstable patient with a tension pneumothorax. Consult medical direction and/or adhere to locally established protocols regarding fluid resuscitation in these patients.

If the mechanism of injury suggests potential spinal injury, full spinal immobilization will be necessary. Blunt trauma to the chest, especially if the force is great enough, can cause injury to the cervical or thoracic spine.

Prompt transport to a trauma center is essential in the emergency care of the patient with a tension pneumothorax. Notify the receiving facility as early as possible so that the appropriate resources (eg, surgery) can be allocated.

Table 3-7 Emergency Care for a Tension Pneumothorax

Ensure a patent airway.
Provide 100% supplemental oxygen or ventilatory support as needed.
Perform a needle thoracentesis to evacuate air from the pleural space.
If internal hemorrhage is suspected, start two large-bore IV lines and infuse fluids to maintain adequate perfusion. Consult with medical control as needed.
Fully immobilize the patient's spine if the mechanism of injury suggests spinal trauma.
Promptly transport the patient to a trauma center with early notification of the patient's condition and your estimated time of arrival.

Summary

Blunt or penetrating trauma to the chest can result in a variety of injuries, including, among others, open pneumothorax, tension pneumothorax, myocardial contusion, pericardial tamponade, and disruption of the great vessels.

The patient in this case study had an open pneumothorax (sucking chest wound) that was sealed with an occlusive dressing. As time progressed, the patient's condition deteriorated. This was the result of a tension pneumothorax—pressure increased within the pleural space, compromising the cardiovascular and respiratory systems. Fortunately, simply lifting a corner of the occlusive dressing improved the patient's condition. However, this is not always the case.

Cardiac arrest secondary to thoracic trauma carries a very high mortality rate. This reinforces the importance of a careful, systematic assessment of the patient in order to detect life-threatening injuries and begin immediate treatment before cardiac arrest occurs.

Emergency care for the victim of a tension pneumothorax focuses on ensuring adequate oxygenation and ventilation by administering 100% supplemental oxygen or assisting ventilations, immobilizing the spine if the mechanism of injury suggests spinal trauma, and performing a needle thoracentesis to relieve pressure in the pleural space, thus allowing the lung to reexpand and participate in the exchange of oxygen and carbon dioxide. Refer to locally established protocols to determine if needle thoracentesis is within your EMS system's scope of practice for your level of certification.

IV fluid boluses of normal saline or lactated ringers (20 mL/kg) may be needed to maintain perfusion if internal hemorrhage is suspected. Consult with medical control as needed regarding fluid resuscitation in the patient with a tension pneumothorax.

4

40-Year-Old Male Who Was the Victim of an Assault

Law enforcement requests your assistance at a residence at 556 North Wagonwheel Drive for a 40-year-old male who was assaulted. The time of call is 2:15 AM, and your response time to the scene is approximately 8 minutes.

1. What should you consider when responding to the scene of this call?

_____

_____

_____

_____

Three police officers are at the scene when you and your partner arrive. The suspect has been apprehended and is in police custody. You find the patient lying supine in the front yard of the residence. His shirt was torn off during the assault, and his pants have dried blood stains on them. As you approach him, you immediately note a large area of bruising across his abdomen.

You introduce yourself to the patient, who is conscious and alert, and perform an initial assessment **(Table 4-1)**. Your partner opens the jump kit and prepares to administer oxygen to the patient.

Table 4-1 Initial Assessment

Mechanism of Injury	Blunt abdominal trauma
Level of Consciousness	Conscious but restless; alert to person, place, and time
Chief Complaint	"Mike hit me in the back of the head. When I fell to the ground, he started kicking me in the stomach. My belly is killing me!"
Airway and Breathing	Airway is patent, respirations are increased with adequate tidal volume.
Circulation	Pulse is strong and rapid, no active bleeding is noted, skin is cool and moist.

2. What injury or injuries should you suspect based on the mechanism of injury described by the patient?

_____

_____

_____

_____

While your partner maintains manual stabilization of the patient's head, you apply 100% supplemental oxygen via a nonrebreathing mask. Your partner asks the patient about the dried blood on his pants. The patient replies, "Well, I actually started the fight by hitting Mike in the face. When he was kicking me in the stomach, blood from his nose must have dripped on my pants." Because of the potential for multiple systems trauma, you perform a rapid trauma assessment **(Table 4-2)**.

Table 4-2 Rapid Trauma Assessment

Head	Hematoma to the back of the head, no bleeding is present.
Neck	Trachea is midline, jugular veins are normal, no cervical spine deformities.
Chest	No obvious trauma to the chest, chest wall is symmetrical, breath sounds are clear and equal bilaterally to auscultation.
Abdomen/Pelvis	Diffuse bruising to the abdomen, abdomen is nondistended, palpable tenderness to the right upper abdominal quadrant, pelvis is stable.
Lower Extremities	No obvious trauma, perfusion and sensory/motor function are grossly intact.
Upper Extremities	No obvious trauma, perfusion and sensory/motor function are grossly intact.
Posterior	Several small abrasions to the lower back, no active bleeding

You and your partner agree that because of the signs of shock the patient is experiencing (i.e., restlessness, tachycardia, tachypnea, clammy skin), as well as the obvious abdominal bruising, that immediate transport to the hospital is indicated. You immobilize the patient's spine with a cervical collar and long spine board and then load him into the ambulance. Once inside, you obtain baseline vital signs and a SAMPLE history (Table 4-3).

Table 4-3 Baseline Vital Signs and SAMPLE History

Blood Pressure	100/60 mm Hg
Pulse	118 beats/min and regular, weaker than before
Respirations	24 breaths/min, adequate tidal volume
Oxygen Saturation	97% (on 100% oxygen)
Signs and Symptoms	Abdominal bruising and pain, hematoma to the back of the head, signs of shock
Allergies	"I'm allergic to codeine."
Medications	"I take one aspirin a day."
Pertinent Past History	"Not that I am aware of. My doctor told me to take one aspirin a day to prevent a heart attack."
Last Oral Intake	"We ate pizza about an hour ago."
Events Leading to the Injury	"Mike and I got into a fight over a poker hand, which is when I clocked him."

3. What is the etiology of this patient's shock?

_____

_____

_____

_____

You begin transport to a trauma center and establish two IV lines of normal saline with 16-gauge catheters while en route. Because the patient's blood pressure is relatively stable and he is conscious and alert, you set the flow rate on the IVs to keep the vein open for the time being. Additionally, you apply a cardiac monitor and assess the patient's cardiac rhythm (Figure 4-1).

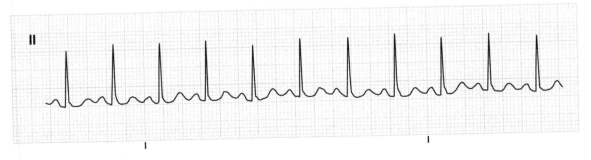

■ **Figure 4-1** Your patient's cardiac rhythm.

4. How could this patient's medication (aspirin) affect his condition?

_____

_____

_____

_____

During transport, you note a drop in the patient's blood pressure, which is now 90/50 mm Hg. While you are infusing 20 ml/kg of normal saline, you perform a detailed physical examination of the patient **(Table 4-4)**, who remains conscious, although more restless.

Table 4-4 Detailed Physical Examination

Head and Face	No obvious trauma to the scalp; ears, nose, and mouth are clear; pupils appear dilated and are sluggishly reactive to light.
Neck	Jugular veins appear flat, trachea is midline.
Chest	No obvious trauma to the chest, chest wall is symmetrical, breath sounds are clear and equal bilaterally to auscultation.
Abdomen/Pelvis	Diffuse bruising to the abdomen, abdomen is rigid and distended, palpable tenderness to the right upper abdominal quadrant, pelvis is stable.
Lower Extremities	No obvious trauma, sensory/motor function is grossly intact, pedal pulses are weakly palpable.
Upper Extremities	No obvious trauma, sensory/motor function is grossly intact, radial pulses are weakly palpable.
Posterior	Examined in the rapid trauma assessment. Patient is immobilized to long spine board.

5. What findings in the detailed examination indicate that your patient is deteriorating?

_____

_____

_____

_____

With an estimated time of arrival to the trauma center of approximately 12 minutes, you continue to administer normal saline fluid boluses of 20 ml/kg. After performing an ongoing assessment **(Table 4-5)**, you call your radio report to the receiving facility.

Table 4-5 Ongoing Assessment

Level of Consciousness	Conscious, more restless
Airway and Breathing	Airway remains patent; respirations, 24 breaths/min with adequate tidal volume.
Oxygen Saturation	96% (on 100% oxygen)
Blood Pressure	96/56 mm Hg
Pulse	100 beats/min, regular and stronger
ECG	Sinus tachycardia

6. What role do IV crystalloid solutions play in shock management?

_____

_____

_____

_____

Upon arrival at the emergency department, a diagnostic peritoneal lavage (DPL) is performed and is positive for blood in the intraabdominal cavity. Following additional stabilization in the emergency department, the patient is taken to surgery, where a laceration to the liver was found and bleeding was controlled. After spending 12 days in the hospital, the patient was discharged home.

1. What should you consider when responding to the scene of this call?

Your foremost concern should be the safety of you and your partner. At this point, you have received no information regarding the safety of the scene. The presence of law enforcement does not automatically make the scene secure. Prior to entering this potentially volatile environment, you must contact the on-scene police officer and determine if the scene is safe for you to enter.

Your primary responsibility as a paramedic is to yourself. This should not be confused with your primary duty, which is to provide safe and effective emergency care to the patient. Once you have determined that you are safe, the safety of your partner, the patient, and any bystanders (in that order) should come next. Likewise, your partner should be doing the same.

2. What injury or injuries should you suspect based on the mechanism of injury described by the patient?

The abdominal bruising is an obvious sign of trauma, which should be assumed to be a manifestation of intraabdominal bleeding. However, this patient was also struck in the back of the head. Although he is conscious and alert at the present time, do not discount the possibility of serious head trauma. Injuries such as subdural hematomas, which result from slow venous bleeding in the cranium, may not present with signs and symptoms for days or weeks.

Because you do not know the force with which the patient was struck in the head, you should also assume spinal injury until proven otherwise. The paramedic must always perform a careful, systematic assessment of the patient with possible multiple body systems trauma. It is often the least obvious injuries that are the most life threatening.

3. What is the etiology of this patient's shock?

It is likely that this patient is in hemorrhagic shock (hypoperfusion) from internal bleeding within the abdominal cavity. Palpable pain to the right upper abdominal quadrant suggests injury to the liver. However, because the bruising is diffuse, injury to the spleen, which is located in the left upper abdominal quadrant, is also possible.

The spleen and liver are the two solid organs in the upper quadrants of the true (anterior) abdominal cavity **(Figure 4-2)**. In contrast to hollow organs (eg, stomach, gallbladder), which, when injured, spill their contents into the abdominal cavity and cause peritonitis (inflammation of the abdominal cavity lining), solid organs often bleed profusely when injured.

This patient is already demonstrating signs of shock, which is likely the result of injury to the liver. The liver contains approximately 40% of a person's total blood volume at any given time and is highly vascular. Because it is the largest organ in the abdominal cavity, the liver is especially prone to injury following blunt trauma to the abdomen. Liver injury is common following trauma to the eighth through twelfth ribs on the right side.

Because of the broad spectrum of possible injuries to multiple organs, abdominal trauma is often difficult to evaluate in the prehospital setting. The paramedic, when evaluating the victim of abdominal trauma, should maintain a high index of suspicion for intraabdominal bleeding, especially when the patient is exhibiting signs of shock. In fact, when a trauma patient presents with signs of shock but no external signs of injury, the paramedic should suspect intraabdominal bleeding. The retroperitoneal space, which lies behind the true abdomen, is a common source for hidden bleeding and may not present with typical external signs of intraabdominal bleeding, such as abdominal bruising, distention, and rigidity.

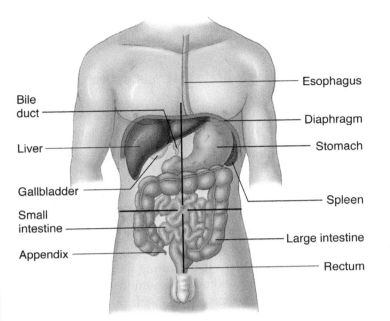

Bile duct

Liver

Gallbladder

Small intestine

Appendix

Esophagus

Diaphragm

Stomach

Spleen

Large intestine

Rectum

■ **Figure 4-2**
Solid organs, such as the liver and spleen, often bleed profusely when injured.

Large lacerations to the liver can rapidly cause death due to exsanguination, whereas smaller liver lacerations may take longer to present with signs of shock. This underscores the importance of a close examination of the mechanism of injury in patients with abdominal trauma.

Rapid identification and treatment of shock and prompt transport for surgical intervention is clearly more important than trying to determine the exact site of the intraabdominal injury. Definitive care for internal bleeding cannot be provided in the field because surgical access to the site of the bleeding cannot be gained. Most patients who die from abdominal trauma do so because of continuing hemorrhage and delayed surgical repair.

4. How could this patient's medication (aspirin) affect his condition?

Aspirin (acetylsalicylic acid, or ASA) inhibits platelet aggregation by blocking the formation of thromboxane A2. This hinders the body's natural attempts to maintain hemostasis, which is the initial physiologic response of the body following an internal or external wound.

Hemostasis is the process by which bleeding stops. It involves localized vasoconstriction, formation of a platelet "plug," blood coagulation (clotting), and eventually the growth of fibrous tissue into the blood clot. Combined, these processes permanently close and seal the injured vessel.

Under normal circumstances, platelets adhere to injured vessels and to collagen in the connective tissue that surrounds the injured vessel. The platelets then swell, become sticky, and secrete chemicals that activate other surrounding platelets. If thromboxane A2 is blocked, this process would occur much less effectively because the surface of the platelet would lose its ability to adhere to the injured vessel (ie, the platelet would be less sticky) and localized vasoconstriction would be limited. With two key components of the hemostatic process blocked (ie, platelet aggregation and vasoconstriction), the injured vessel or vessels would have an increased tendency to bleed.

Hemostasis is a powerful protective mechanism of the human body that, in combination with prompt recognition and management of internal bleeding and immediate transport, can sustain a patient's life until the injury can be surgically repaired. However, if the patient takes medications that inhibit blood clotting (eg, aspirin, coumadin), hemostasis occurs less efficiently. Clearly, severe external or internal injuries with profuse bleeding are worse in patients taking aspirin or coumadin.

5. What findings in the detailed examination indicate that your patient is deteriorating?

The following detailed physical examination findings, which were not present during the rapid trauma assessment, indicate that your patient's condition is deteriorating:

- **Dilated, sluggishly reactive pupils,** which indicates cerebral hypoxia secondary to worsened shock (hypoperfusion).

- **Flattened jugular veins,** which indicates that the patient's blood volume is decreased secondary to continued intraabdominal bleeding.

- **Rigid, distended abdomen,** which is secondary to increased bleeding within the intraabdominal cavity.

In addition to these abnormal findings, the patient is becoming more restless, his blood pressure has decreased, and his pulse is weaker. These findings clearly indicate that the patient may be entering a state of decompensated shock.

Continuous reassessment of the patient in shock is critical. Deterioration in the patient's condition will require adjustments in management, which, at this point, must be aggressive.

6. What role do IV crystalloid solutions play in shock management?

The goal of managing a patient in shock is to maintain adequate perfusion. In the prehospital setting, this is most effectively accomplished by administering crystalloid IV fluids (eg, normal saline, lactated ringers).

Crystalloid intravenous solutions include normal saline, lactated ringers, and 5% dextrose in water (D_5W). In contrast to colloid solutions, such as whole blood, plasma, or synthetic plasma substitutes (eg, dextran, hespan), crystalloid solutions have smaller molecules and less osmotic pressure. This means that crystalloid solutions equilibrate more rapidly between the vascular and extravascular spaces.

Two-thirds of infused crystalloid solution leaves the vascular space within 1 hour; therefore, you must infuse 3 ml of crystalloid solution for each 1 ml of estimated blood loss.

Glucose-containing crystalloids, such as D_5W, provide immediate but transient (5 to 10 minutes) volume expansion. This is because the glucose rapidly leaves the intravascular space with a resultant increase in the amount of free water. For this reason, D_5W would not be an appropriate choice for IV fluid resuscitation in the patient with shock.

Lactated ringers and normal saline are the preferred crystalloids for fluid resuscitation in shock. They are both well-balanced solutions that contain many of the same chemicals found in human blood.

It is important to remember that IV fluids are used to maintain blood pressure, not increase it. Aggressive fluid resuscitation in uncontrolled hemorrhage (eg, internal bleeding) may exacerbate bleeding by diluting clotting factors and increasing blood pressure, thus interfering with hemostasis. Additionally, crystalloid solutions do not have the ability to carry oxygen. Their exclusive role is to increase the volume in which the formed blood components circulate, thus maintaining tissue perfusion until the patient can be treated definitively. The paramedic should consult with medical control regarding fluid resuscitation for patients with trauma-induced shock.

The mainstays of shock management include maintaining a patent airway, ensuring adequate oxygenation and ventilation, controlling external hemorrhage, rapidly identifying and treating shock, and immediately transporting the patient to a trauma center for definitive care. Unless on-scene time will be unusually lengthy (eg., prolonged extrication), IV therapy and other time-consuming interventions should be performed en route to the hospital.

Summary

In cases where a patient is bleeding externally, management is relatively easy because you can see the source of bleeding and take measures to control it. Internal bleeding, however, is more elusive in that it cannot be controlled in the prehospital setting. Additionally, bleeding within the intraabdominal cavity can be especially problematic because the patient may not present with external signs of abdominal trauma (eg, bruising, rigidity, distention), especially when the source of the bleeding is in the retroperitoneal space. This requires the paramedic to perform a rapid, yet careful assessment of the patient, identify the signs of shock, and promptly transport the patient to a trauma center where surgical intervention can occur. Scene management should be limited to that of addressing immediate life threats only, such as problems with airway, breathing, and circulation. Additional treatment, however, such as IV therapy, should be performed while en route to the hospital. It is important to understand that definitive care cannot be provided outside the hospital, and that regardless of how much time is spent at the scene, you cannot change the travel distance to the hospital.

5

39-Year-Old Male Injured in a House Fire

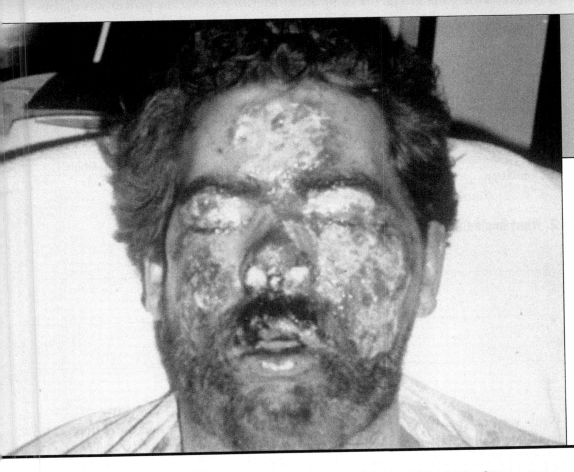

At 5:20 AM, the fire department requests your assistance at the scene of a house fire where they have rescued a 39-year-old male from a burning building. While en route to the scene, the fire commander advises you that the patient is unconscious and has extensive burns. Your response time to the scene is approximately 8 minutes.

1. **What life-threatening conditions should you anticipate based on the information you have received thus far?**

_____

_____

_____

_____

Upon arriving at the scene, you are immediately escorted to the patient. Firefighters have placed a blanket on the patient and have applied 100% supplemental oxygen via a nonrebreathing mask. The fire commander advises you that the patient was unconscious at the time of his rescue. While your partner opens the trauma kit, you perform an initial assessment **(Table 5-1)**.

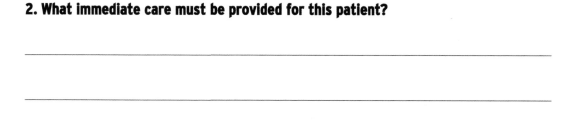

Table 5-1 Initial Assessment

Mechanism of Injury	Trapped in a burning building
Level of Consciousness	Unconscious and unresponsive
Chief Complaint	Unconscious, severe burns, respiratory compromise
Airway and Breathing	Respirations, rapid and labored; stridor is heard on inhalation.
Circulation	Pulse is weak, rapid, and regular; no gross bleeding noted.

2. What immediate care must be provided for this patient?

_____

_____

_____

While your partner is managing the patient's airway, he tells you that the patient's nasal hairs are singed and that there is carbonaceous sputum in his airway. The patient's spine is fully immobilized, and he is rapidly loaded into the ambulance. While your partner and a firefighter prepare to definitively secure the patient's airway, you perform a rapid trauma assessment **(Table 5-2)**.

Table 5-2 Rapid Trauma Assessment

Head	Partial- and full-thickness burns, no deformities or bleeding, singed nasal hair, carbonaceous sputum
Neck	Partial- and full-thickness burns, trachea midline, jugular veins flat, no spinal deformities
Chest	Partial- and full-thickness burns, chest wall stable and symmetrical, breath sounds clear to auscultation bilaterally
Abdomen/Pelvis	Partial- and full-thickness burns, abdomen is soft to palpation, pelvis is stable.
Lower Extremities	No obvious trauma; pedal pulses, weak; unable to assess sensory and motor function (unconscious)
Upper Extremities	Partial- and full-thickness burns; radial pulses, weak; unable to assess sensory and motor function (unconscious)
Posterior	Superficial burns, no spinal deformities

3. What percentage of this patient's body surface area has been burned?

_____

_____

_____

_____

4. Which of this patient's burns are classified as critical burns?

_____

_____

_____

_____

While you are preparing to initiate two large-bore IV lines, a firefighter obtains baseline vital signs and a SAMPLE history **(Table 5-3)**. Because the patient is unconscious, his medical information is unobtainable. Your partner has successfully intubated the patient and is assisting his ventilations. The ECG leads are applied to areas of superficial burns on the patient's shoulder and on his left lower leg. You assess his cardiac rhythm, which reveals sinus tachycardia at a rate of 130 beats/min.

Table 5-3 Baseline Vital Signs and SAMPLE History

Blood Pressure	88/60 mm Hg
Pulse	130 beats/min, weak and regular
Respirations	Intubated, ventilated at 15 breaths/min
Oxygen Saturation	95% (ventilated with 100% oxygen)
Signs and Symptoms	Severe burns to the upper body, respiratory insufficiency, unconscious
Allergies	Unknown
Medications	Unknown
Pertinent Past History	Unknown
Last Oral Intake	Unknown
Events Leading to the Injury	Neighbors reported hearing a small explosion shortly before the house caught on fire.

Because your partner's assistance is needed for appropriate patient care, you ask the firefighter to drive the ambulance. Transport is begun to a trauma center located 9 miles away. While en route, you establish two large-bore IV lines of normal saline.

5. What is the appropriate IV fluid regimen for this patient?

_____

_____

_____

_____

6. How will you care for this patient's burns?

_____

_____

_____

_____

The patient's burns have been appropriately cared for and your partner continues ventilatory support. With an estimated time of arrival at the hospital of less than 5 minutes, you perform an ongoing assessment **(Table 5-4)** and then call your radio report to the receiving facility. The patient remains unconscious and is being ventilated by your partner.

Table 5-4 Ongoing Assessment

Level of Consciousness	Unconscious and unresponsive
Airway and Breathing	Intubated, ventilated at a rate of 15 breaths per minute
Oxygen Saturation	96% (ventilated with 100% oxygen)
Blood Pressure	98/64 mm Hg
Pulse	110 beats/min and regular, stronger radial pulses
ECG	Sinus tachycardia

You arrive at the hospital and are immediately met by the attending physician. Following further stabilization in the emergency department, the patient is transferred by helicopter to a burn center. Despite aggressive hospital treatment, the patient died 3 days later due to massive infection.

5

1. What life-threatening conditions should you anticipate based on the information you have received thus far?

Because this patient was unconscious in a smoke-filled environment for an unknown period of time, he has likely inhaled toxic gases and superheated air or steam. At a minimum, you should be prepared to address the following problems:

- **Airway burns and swelling**
  - The highly vascular soft tissue structures of the upper airway rapidly swell in response to toxic inhalation and/or superheated air or steam. This swelling significantly reduces the size of the airway and impairs effective ventilation and oxygenation.
  - In addition to providing ventilatory support, this patient may require early intubation before his airway becomes inaccessible secondary to swelling. If intubation is unsuccessful or otherwise not possible, a cricothyrotomy will be necessary.

- **Toxic inhalation**
  - Most modern residential structures are constructed using synthetic resins and plastics that release toxic gases when burning. When inhaled, they impair gas exchange in the lungs and at the cellular level. Although many toxic gases are produced during the burning process, the following gases are of particular concern:
    - *Carbon monoxide (CO)* is a colorless, odorless, and tasteless gas that is produced during the incomplete combustion of carbon-containing fuels such as gasoline, oil, and wood. CO binds to hemoglobin 200 to 250 times more readily than oxygen and forms carboxyhemoglobin (COHb). Because CO displaces oxygen from the hemoglobin molecule, the oxygen-carrying capacity of the blood is reduced, thus impairing cellular and tissue oxygenation.
    - *Cyanide* is a by-product of the combustion of nylon and polyurethane. It is a rapidly acting toxin that combines and reacts with ferric ions (Fe^3) of the respiratory enzyme cytochrome oxidase, a key constituent in the process of cellular respiration. The chemical reaction of cyanide in the blood results in severe hypoxia and cellular asphyxia.

- **Thermal burns**
  - Although clearly a life-threatening problem, thermal burns to the body are usually not the cause of death in patients who have been entrapped in a burning building. Such patients typically succumb to cellular anoxia and respiratory failure secondary to toxic inhalation. However, you must still be prepared to address issues such as covering the burns, maintaining body temperature, and replacing lost fluid volume.

2. What immediate care must be provided for this patient?

- **Spinal immobilization**
  - Because the patient is unconscious, trauma cannot be ruled out. Therefore, his spine should be fully immobilized.
    - Manually stabilize the patient's head and use the jaw-thrust technique to open his airway.
    - Ensure that the patient's spine is fully immobilized prior to loading him into the ambulance.

- **Positive-pressure ventilatory support**
  - The patient's respiratory effort is inadequate. His breathing is rapid and labored, which is producing inadequate tidal volume. Passive oxygenation, such as with a nonrebreathing mask, will not suffice.
  - Perform BVM ventilations with 100% oxygen to assist the patient's breathing.

- **Endotracheal intubation**
  - Stridor, which is a high-pitched sound heard on inhalation, indicates supraglottic (upper-airway) obstruction. In the case of this patient, the obstruction is due to edematous soft tissue of the airway—likely a result of the direct inhalation of heat and, potentially, flames.
  - This patient must be intubated as soon as possible. Supraglottic swelling severely obscures the anatomic landmarks that you must visualize for intubation. If the airway is not secured with an ET tube now, a cricothyrotomy will be the only means of establishing a patent airway.

3. What percentage of this patient's body surface area has been burned?

According to the Rule of Nines **(Figure 5-1)**, this patient has burns that cover approximately 45 percent of his body surface area (BSA). This patient's burns are summarized, by body region, in **Table 5-5**.

Table 5-5 Calculation of This Patient's Burns

Head, face, and neck: 9%
Anterior trunk (chest and abdomen): 18%
Both upper extremities: 18%

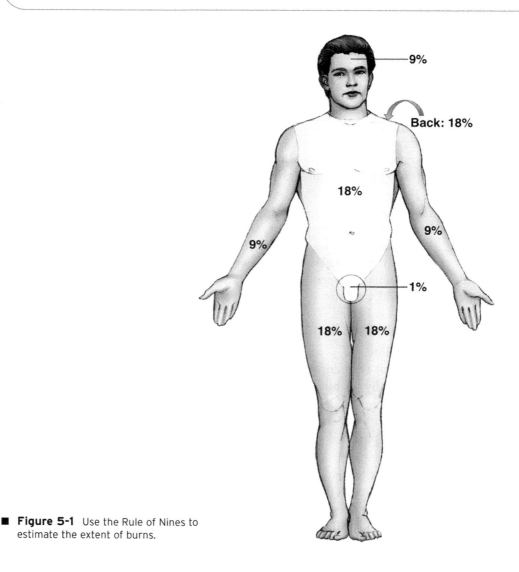

■ **Figure 5-1** Use the Rule of Nines to estimate the extent of burns.

Case Study 5: Answers and Summary

Table 5-6 Burn Severity Classification in Adults

Critical burns
- Burns involving the hands, feet, face, airway, or genitalia
- Full-thickness burns covering more than 10% of the patient's BSA
- Partial-thickness burns covering more than 30% of the patient's BSA
- Burns associated with airway injury (smoke inhalation)
- Burns complicated by significant injuries (eg, fractures, head trauma)

Moderate burns
- Full-thickness burns involving 2% to 10% of the patient's BSA
- Partial-thickness burns covering 15% to 30% of the patient's BSA
- Superficial burns covering more than 50% of the patient's BSA
- No burns of the hands, feet, face, airway, or genitalia

Minor burns
- Full-thickness burns covering less than 2% of the patient's BSA
- Partial-thickness burns covering less than 15% of the patient's BSA
- Superficial burns covering less than 50% of the patient's BSA
- No burns of the hands, feet, face, airway, or genitalia

The Rule of Palms, an alternate method for approximating the extent of a burn, uses the palmar surface of the patient's hand as a point of comparison in gauging the size of the affected BSA. The patient's palm (the hand less the fingers) represents approximately 1 percent of the patient's BSA. By visualizing the palmar surface area and comparing it with the burned area(s), you can obtain a rough estimate of the BSA affected.

Although the percentage of BSA burned is an important calculation to make, it is far more important to determine the location and depth (degree) of the burns. This will give the receiving facility a better idea as to the criticality of the patient's condition.

4. Which of this patient's burns are classified as critical burns?

All of this patient's burns are classified as critical burns. He has burns involving the airway and hands, partial-thickness burns that cover more than 30 percent of his BSA, and full-thickness burns that cover more than 10 percent of his BSA. **Table 5-6** classifies burns by severity in the adult patient.

5. What is the appropriate IV fluid regimen for this patient?

For patients with extensive burns, aggressive IV fluid therapy will be required. Although hypovolemia typically occurs later and is caused when proteins, fluid, and electrolytes migrate into the burned areas, early and aggressive IV fluid therapy can effectively decrease the negative impact of this fluid migration and subsequent profound fluid loss.

After establishing two large-bore IV lines of normal saline (preferably in nonburned areas), administer 20 mL/kg boluses of an isotonic crystalloid to maintain adequate perfusion in the hypotensive patient. During lengthy (greater than 1 hour) transport times, medical control may order you to administer IV fluids based on the Parkland formula. The Parkland formula recommends giving 4 mL of normal saline for each kilogram of body weight, multiplied by the percentage of BSA burned:

$$4 \text{ mL} \times \textbf{Patient weight in kilograms} \times \textbf{BSA burned} = \textbf{Total fluid in 24 hours}$$

Thus, for a 75-kg patient with 45 percent BSA burned, the calculation is as follows:

$$4 \text{ (mL)} \times 75 \text{ (kg)} \times 45 \text{ (BSA)} = \textbf{13,500 mL during the first 24 hours}$$

The Parkland formula further states that the patient should receive half of this amount of fluid (6,750 mL) in the first 8 hours following the burn.

If your transport time is short (less than 1 hour), an initial IV fluid bolus of 0.5 mL for each kilogram of body weight multiplied by the percentage of BSA burned is acceptable and may need to be repeated once or twice within the first hour of care:

0.5 mL × Patient weight in kilograms × BSA burned = Amount of fluid

Thus, for a 75-kg patient with 45 percent BSA burned, the calculation is as follows:

0.5 (mL) × 75 (kg) × 45 (BSA) = 1,688 mL

6. How will you care for this patient's burns?

Dry sterile dressings or a sterile burn pad should be placed on the patient's burns. With this particular patient, it would be best to completely wrap him in a sterile burn sheet as well as a blanket. This will protect against contamination of the burned areas as well as maintain the patient's body temperature. Severe burns disrupt the body's ability to regulate core temperature. As plasma and other body fluids seep into the burned areas, they are evaporated away, which rapidly removes heat energy. This causes rapid heat loss and severe hypothermia.

Infection is a persistent killer of patients with severe burns; however, it may not occur for several days following the burn. Nonetheless, to reduce the patient's exposure to infection, use sterile dressings and avoid gross contamination of all burned areas.

Of the different burn classifications **(Figure 5-2)**, partial-thickness burns that cover greater than 30% BSA and full-thickness burns that cover greater than 10% BSA are associated with the greatest risk of hypovolemia, hypothermia, and infection.

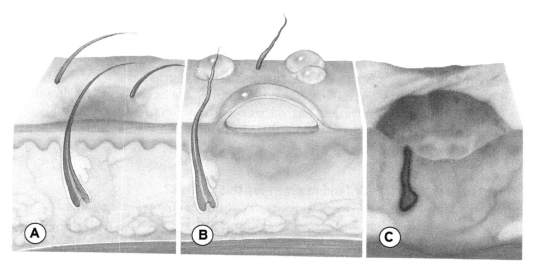

■ **Figure 5-2** Classification of burns.
(A.) Superficial (first-degree) burns involve only the epidermis. The skin turns red but does not blister or actually burn through. (B.) Partial-thickness (second-degree) burns involve some of the dermis, but they do not destroy the entire thickness of the skin. The skin is mottled, white to red, and is often blistered. (C.) Full-thickness (third-degree) burns extend through all layers of the skin and may involve subcutaneous tissue and muscle. The skin is dry, leathery, and often either white or charred.

Remove any potentially restricting items, such as rings, watches, bracelets, or necklaces. Because of his extensive burns, edema may cause this jewelry to act as a tourniquet and occlude arterial blood flow to distal areas. Blisters that form from partial thickness burns should not be ruptured, because this increases the risk of hypovolemia and infection. Never apply burn creams or ointments to the burn. These are of no value in the prehospital setting and will only have to be removed at the hospital.

Summary

Burns account for over 100,000 deaths per year. A burn occurs when the body, or a part of the body, receives more energy than it can absorb without sustaining injury.

Burns are classified as being either superficial (first degree), partial thickness (second degree), or full thickness (third degree).

Patient mortality and morbidity depends on a variety of factors, including the degree of burn, percentage of BSA involved, the patient's age and general health, associated injury, and whether toxic inhalation occurred.

Immediate death from fire is typically the result of toxic gas inhalation (eg, carbon monoxide, cyanide) or swelling and closure of the airway. This is especially true when the patient is trapped and unconscious in a smoke-filled environment. Although the most obvious, the thermal burn injury itself is usually not what kills the patient. Many patients survive the immediate effects of the burn only to succumb to massive infection within a few days to a week.

Immediate care for the burn patient involves removing the patient from the burn environment, which is typically carried out by fire suppression and rescue personnel. Never attempt to rescue a trapped patient by entering a burning building unless you are properly trained, appropriately equipped, and assigned to do so by the incident commander.

Once the patient has been moved to safety, stop the burning process and remove any smoldering clothing by cutting it from around the burned areas. Do not pull adhered clothing from the patient's skin because this will cause additional tissue damage.

Assess the patient's airway and provide 100% oxygen by a nonrebreathing mask or assisted ventilations, depending on the adequacy of the patient's breathing. Be prepared to perform early intubation to protect the airway from swelling.

Care for the partial-thickness and full-thickness burns includes covering them with dry, sterile dressings or a sterile burn sheet. Cover the patient with a blanket to help prevent hypothermia. Consider analgesic medications (eg, Morphine) for pain if the patient is conscious and hemodynamically stable.

Maintain adequate perfusion in the hypotensive patient with 20 mL/kg boluses of an isotonic crystalloid. Use the Parkland formula or other approved IV fluid resuscitation protocol as dictated by your transport time and medical control.

Transport immediately to an appropriate facility, which should be a Level I trauma center or a specialized burn center. Follow locally established protocols regarding transport destination of the severely burned patient. Notify the receiving facility early so that the appropriate resources can be allocated.

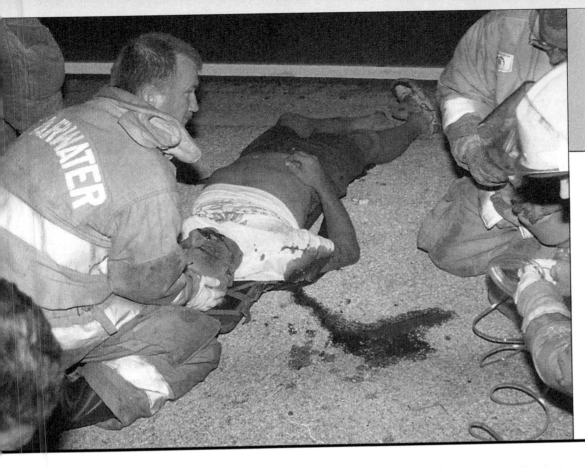

6

50-Year-Old Male with Multiple Injuries

At 3:45 AM, your unit is dispatched to mile marker 540 on Interstate Highway 10 for a 50-year-old male who sustained injuries after being carjacked. While you are en route, an on-scene police officer radios you and advises you that the scene is secure.

You arrive at the scene. Fire personnel are maintaining manual stabilization of the patient's head. Apparently, the patient picked up a hitchhiker who stabbed him several times before pushing him from the slow-moving vehicle. You approach the patient, who is conscious and talking, and perform an initial assessment **(Table 6-1)**.

Table 6-1 Initial Assessment

Mechanism of Injury	Stabbed and pushed from a slow-moving vehicle
Level of Consciousness	Conscious but restless
Chief Complaint	"My chest and hips are killing me!"
Airway and Breathing	Airway is patent; respirations, increased with adequate tidal volume.
Circulation	Radial pulse, weak and rapid; bleeding is noted from a large laceration to the upper left arm and from a stab wound to the left anterior chest; skin is pale, cool, and clammy.

1. What immediate care is required for this patient?

_____

_____

_____

_____

Fire personnel have retrieved a cervical collar, spine board, and straps from the ambulance. After completing the initial care of the patient, you perform a rapid trauma assessment (Table 6-2). The patient remains conscious and is talking to your partner.

Table 6-2 Rapid Trauma Assessment

Head	Several small scalp lacerations, no active bleeding, no deformities or depressions to the skull
Neck	Trachea is midline; jugular veins appear distended; no cervical spine deformities.
Chest	Single stab wound to the left anterior chest (sealed), multiple abrasions to the anterior chest, chest wall is stable to palpation, breath sounds are clear and equal bilaterally.
Abdomen/Pelvis	Abdomen is soft and nontender without bruising, rigidity, or distention; pain to the pelvis upon palpation.
Lower Extremities	Multiple abrasions, motor and sensory functions are grossly intact, pedal pulses are bilaterally absent.
Upper Extremities	Multiple abrasions, laceration to upper right arm (bleeding controlled), motor and sensory functions are grossly intact, radial pulses are bilaterally weak.
Posterior	The patient is not log rolled due to the pelvic pain; however, no obvious posterior bleeding is noted.

2. What does jugular venous distention in this patient suggest?

_____

_____

_____

_____

Upon completion of the rapid trauma assessment of the patient, a cervical collar is applied. Because he is experiencing pain to his pelvis, he is placed onto the long spine board with an orthopedic (scoop) stretcher. After fully immobilizing the patient's spine, you quickly load him into the ambulance. Your partner obtains baseline vital signs and a SAMPLE history (Table 6-3) while you prepare to initiate IV therapy.

Table 6-3 Baseline Vital Signs and SAMPLE History

Blood Pressure	90/60 mm Hg
Pulse	118 beats/min and regular, weak at the radial artery
Respirations	24 breaths/min, adequate tidal volume
Oxygen Saturation	96% (on 100% oxygen)
Signs and Symptoms	Laceration to the upper right arm, stab wound to the left anterior chest, pelvic pain, hypotension, tachycardia, jugular venous distention
Allergies	No known drug allergies
Medications	None
Pertinent Past History	Appendectomy 10 years ago
Last Oral Intake	Supper, approximately 8 hours ago
Events Leading to the Injury	"I picked up a hitchhiker. We were only traveling about 20 miles per hour when he stabbed me and then pushed me out of the car."

After establishing two large-bore IV lines of normal saline, transport is begun to a trauma center located 8 miles away. En route, you apply a cardiac monitor and assess the patient's cardiac rhythm **(Figure 6-1)**.

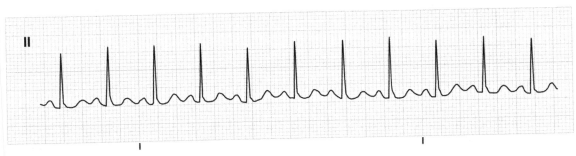

■ Figure 6-1 Your patient's cardiac rhythm.

3. What additional signs may accompany jugular venous distention in a patient with penetrating chest trauma?

_____

_____

_____

_____

4. What specific treatment is required to treat this patient's condition?

_____

_____

_____

_____

_____

Because the estimated time of arrival at the hospital is less than 5 minutes, you are unable to conduct a detailed physical exam, so you quickly perform an ongoing assessment **(Table 6-4)** and then call your radio report to the receiving facility.

Table 6-4 Ongoing Assessment

Level of Consciousness	Conscious, increasing restlessness
Airway and Breathing	Airway remains patent; respirations, 26 breaths/min with adequate tidal volume.
Oxygen Saturation	96% (on 100% oxygen)
Blood Pressure	80/66 mm Hg
Pulse	130 beats/min, weak and regular
ECG	Sinus tachycardia

You provide aggressive IV fluid resuscitation and continuous monitoring throughout transport. Upon arrival at the hospital, the physician assesses the patient and confirms a pericardial tamponade. An immediate pericardiocentesis is performed, after which the patient's blood pressure and clinical condition improve. He is taken to surgery, where his injury is repaired. A subsequent radiograph of the patient's pelvis reveals no fractures.

1. What immediate care is required for this patient?

This patient has multiple significant mechanisms of injury. Each one must be addressed based on severity (ie, what will kill the patient first). Continue to have the firefighter maintain manual stabilization of the patient's head while you and your partner perform the following interventions:

- **Control external hemorrhage**
  - All external bleeding must be stopped immediately. Your partner can accomplish this while you tend to the patient's airway.
    - The stab wound to the left anterior chest should be covered with an occlusive dressing. Any open wound to the chest could indicate underlying pulmonary injury and an open pneumothorax (sucking chest wound).

- **100% supplemental oxygen**
  - Although increased, this patient's respiratory effort is adequate (good tidal volume); therefore, 100% supplemental oxygen via a nonrebreathing mask should be applied.
    - Monitor this patient's respiratory effort carefully and be prepared to initiate positive-pressure ventilatory support if his breathing becomes inadequate (eg, reduced tidal volume, profoundly labored).

Teamwork between you and your partner is critical to providing effective patient care. Had the firefighters not been present to assist with spinal immobilization (meaning that your partner would have to), your first priority would have been to control the external bleeding. Only after the external bleeding is controlled would you apply oxygen. You must treat injuries in the order of what is going to kill the patient *first*. Severe external bleeding can cause death within a few seconds if not immediately controlled. Delaying oxygen therapy for the 1 or 2 minutes that it takes to control the severe bleeding will not kill the patient.

2. What does jugular venous distention in this patient suggest?

The stab wound to the left side of the chest and jugular venous distention should make you suspicious of a *pericardial tamponade*. The presence of bilaterally equal breath sounds rules out a tension pneumothorax, another potential cause of jugular venous distention.

The heart is encased in a fibrous, inelastic membrane called the pericardium. The pericardial space, which is actually a potential space that normally contains 20 to 30 mL of lubricating fluid, exists between the pericardium and the heart. Blood can enter the pericardial space if small myocardial blood vessels (eg, coronary arteries) are torn or if direct penetration of the myocardium occurs. As a result, a condition called hemopericardium occurs. As more blood enters the pericardial space, a pericardial tamponade can develop **(Figure 6-2)**.

Pericardial tamponade is most commonly associated with stab wounds to the chest. Larger penetrating injuries, such as gunshot wounds, often create a large enough hole in the pericardium for blood to exit the pericardial space and are typically associated with exsanguination into the thoracic cavity rather than pericardial tamponade.

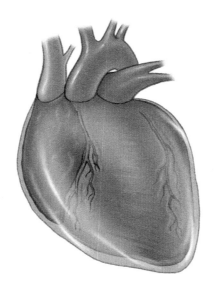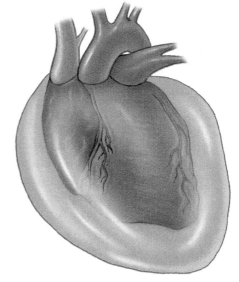

■ **Figure 6-2** Pericardial tamponade occurs when blood or other fluids accumulate in the pericardial sac. As bleeding into the pericardium continues, the myocardium is compressed, which impairs venous return and cardiac output.

Because the tough, fibrous pericardium does not stretch, accumulating blood puts pressure on the heart, affecting both the systolic and diastolic phases of the cardiac cycle. Pressure on the heart impairs venous return to the heart (preload) and limits right ventricular filling. As venous pressure increases, the jugular veins become distended.

3. What additional signs may accompany jugular venous distention in a patient with penetrating chest trauma?

In the adult patient, the pericardial space can hold 200 to 300 mL of blood before signs of a pericardial tamponade become evident; however, smaller volumes of blood can still significantly reduce cardiac output. Progression of a pericardial tamponade depends on how fast blood is filling the pericardial space.

As previously discussed, pericardial tamponade causes an increase in venous pressure and jugular venous distention. In addition, right ventricular expansion (and filling) is impaired, which compromises output through the pulmonary arteries and subsequent venous return to the left side of the heart. This causes a *decreased cardiac output and systemic hypotension*. A *reflex tachycardia* attempts to (but cannot) compensate for the low cardiac output state.

Because myocardial contractility is compromised, the patient's systolic blood pressure decreases. Additionally, decreased ability of the myocardium to fully relax causes an increase in the diastolic blood pressure. This results in a *narrowed pulse pressure* (the difference between the systolic and diastolic blood pressure).

Pulsus paradoxus, which is characterized by a drop in systolic blood pressure of greater than 10 mm Hg during inspiration, may also occur and is caused when the expanding lungs literally stop the heart in animation by putting additional pressure on the already compressed myocardium. Pulsus paradoxus can be determined clinically by noting a diminished or even disappearing radial pulse upon inspiration.

Increasing amounts of blood in the pericardium may also cause *muffled or distant heart sounds*; however, this is often difficult to hear, especially in a loud environment such as the back of a moving ambulance.

Beck's triad, a classic finding in pericardial tamponade, is characterized by three clinical signs: (1) jugular venous distention, (2) muffled heart sounds, and (3) a narrowing pulse pressure. However, all three of these clinical signs may not be present, especially if the patient is hypovolemic from other injuries (eg, pelvic fracture), which is possible in this patient because of his pelvic pain. The physical findings of a pericardial tamponade are summarized in **Table 6-5**.

Table 6-5 Physical Findings of a Pericardial Tamponade

Tachycardia and hypotension
Bilaterally equal breath sounds
Midline trachea
Beck's triad
• Jugular venous distention
• Muffled or distant heart sounds
• Narrowing pulse pressure

4. What specific treatment is required to treat this patient's condition?

Patients with pericardial tamponade require rapid transport to a trauma center with continuous monitoring of airway, breathing, and circulation en route. As with any critical trauma patient, unnecessary delays must not occur in the field.

Treatment for patients with pericardial tamponade includes removing blood from the pericardium by a procedure called *pericardiocentesis.* This procedure, however, is almost exclusively performed in the emergency department and is only a temporizing intervention until bleeding control and surgical repair of the injury can occur in the operating room. Refer to locally established protocols in regards to performing pericardiocentesis in the prehospital setting.

Prehospital management begins by ensuring airway patency and administering 100% supplemental oxygen. If the patient's respiratory effort is inadequate (eg, reduced tidal volume), assisted ventilations with 100% oxygen will be necessary.

Perform spinal immobilization if the mechanism of injury suggests spinal trauma. Because this patient was pushed out of a moving vehicle, he will clearly require immobilization.

Crystalloid IV fluids should be administered to increase venous return to the right atrium (preload). By increasing preload, the full and vigorously contracting atrium will force blood into the ventricles, thus stretching its walls. Stretching of the ventricular wall enhances contractility and the force with which it ejects blood out to the body. Increased cardiac contractility due to stretching of the myocardial wall is called the *Frank-Starling mechanism;* which, by administering IV fluids, will be enhanced, and can maintain cardiac output until a pericardiocentesis can be performed.

Continuous cardiac monitoring is essential in the management of a patient with pericardial tamponade. Decreased cardiac output and hypoperfusion can result in life-threatening dysrhythmias. Pericardial tamponade is also associated with pulseless electrical activity (PEA), a condition in which a cardiac rhythm is present on the cardiac monitor but a palpable pulse is not present.

Management for the patient with a pericardial tamponade is summarized in **Table 6-6**.

Table 6-6 Management for a Pericardial Tamponade

Ensure airway patency • Immobilize the spine if the mechanism of injury suggests spinal trauma.
Administer 100% supplemental oxygen • Assist ventilations with 100% oxygen if the patient is breathing inadequately.
Establish two large-bore IV lines • Infuse isotonic crystalloids to increase preload and maintain cardiac output.
Continuous cardiac monitoring • Be alert for cardiac dysrhythmias or cardiac arrest (PEA).
Rapid transport to a trauma center • Notify the receiving facility early. • Reassess the patient frequently while en route.

Summary

Pericardial tamponade is a condition in which blood accumulates in the pericardium and causes hemodynamic compromise. It is most often the result of penetrating trauma, specifically stab wounds to the chest. A small tear in a myocardial blood vessel or direct penetrating trauma to the myocardium causes blood to seep into the myocardium, which puts pressure on the heart and impairs its performance. The progression of a pericardial tamponade depends on the rate at which blood is accumulating within the pericardium.

Patients with pericardial tamponade typically present with signs of shock (eg, tachycardia, hypotension, diaphoresis) as well as jugular venous distention, muffled heart sounds, and a narrowing pulse pressure (Beck's triad). If the patient is severely hypovolemic from other injuries, however, jugular venous distention may not be present.

Complications associated with pericardial tamponade include cardiac dysrhythmias, such as ventricular fibrillation or ventricular tachycardia, or cardiac arrest with PEA.

A careful, systematic assessment of the patient is required to identify the signs of pericardial tamponade and initiate the most appropriate treatment. Prehospital management consists of ensuring a patent airway, administering 100% oxygen (or ventilatory support if needed), immobilizing the spine if the mechanism of injury suggests spinal trauma, infusing IV crystalloids to increase venous return, and rapidly transporting the patient to a trauma center. Cardiac monitoring en route is essential in being able to identify and treat life-threatening cardiac dysrhythmias.

A pericardiocentesis is required to remove blood from the pericardium, thus improving cardiac output. However, this is almost exclusively performed in the emergency department by a physician and is only a temporizing intervention until the injury can be repaired surgically.

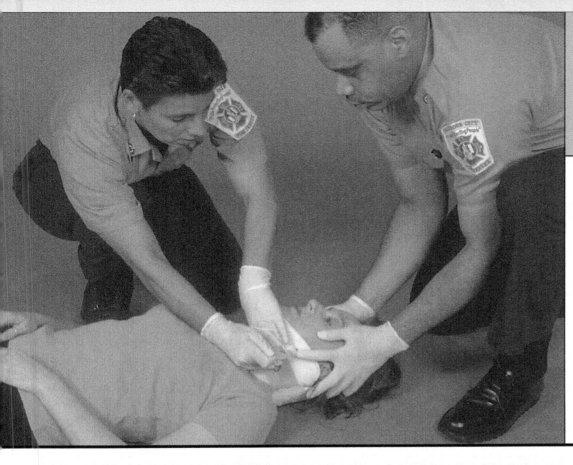

7

30-Year-Old Female with Spine Trauma

At 12:50 PM, you receive a call to 114 East Yolanda Street for a 30-year-old female with back pain following a fall. Your response time to the scene is less than 5 minutes.

Upon arriving at the scene, you find the patient lying supine in the deep end of an empty swimming pool. She is being tended to be a neighbor. According to the patient, she was cleaning the deck around her pool, preparing to put water in it, when she slipped on some leaves and fell into the deep end of the pool. Your partner initiates manual in-line stabilization of the patient's head while you perform an initial assessment **(Table 7-1)**.

Table 7-1 Initial Assessment

Mechanism of Injury	Fall
Level of Consciousness	Conscious and alert to person, place, and time
Chief Complaint	Pain in the middle of the back, tingling in the legs
Airway and Breathing	Airway is patent; respirations, normal rate and depth.
Circulation	Radial pulse, normal rate and strong; skin, warm and dry; no bleeding is present.

1. What common mechanisms of injury cause spinal trauma?

_____

_____

_____

_____

You apply 100% supplemental oxygen to the patient via a nonrebreathing mask. She denies a loss of consciousness before and after the fall, stating that she merely slipped on the leaves and fell. After palpating the cervical spine and confirming the absence of swelling or deformities, you apply a cervical collar and then perform a focused physical examination based on the patient's chief complaint **(Table 7-2)**.

Table 7-2 Focused Physical Examination

Inspection	Large abrasion to the midthoracic region of the spine with swelling, no deformities noted, no obvious bleeding
Palpation	No crepitus noted upon palpation, point tenderness to the area of the sixth thoracic vertebrae
Skin	Warm and dry above and below the site of injury
Neurologic	Pedal pulses are present bilaterally; tingling to both lower extremities; gross motor function is present bilaterally.

2. What are the specific types of spinal cord injury?

_____

_____

_____

_____

After completing the focused examination, the patient's spine is fully immobilized. The patient is then placed into the ambulance. You obtain baseline vital signs and a SAMPLE history **(Table 7-3)** while your partner moves to the driver's seat.

Table 7-3 Baseline Vital Signs and SAMPLE History

Blood Pressure	116/78 mm Hg
Pulse	84 beats/min, strong and regular
Respirations	16 breaths/min, adequate tidal volume
Oxygen Saturation	99% (on 100% oxygen)
Signs and Symptoms	Abrasions and swelling to the thoracic area of the spinal column, tingling in the lower extremities
Allergies	Penicillin
Medications	Birth control pills
Pertinent Past History	None
Last Oral Intake	Lunch, approximately 1 hour ago
Events Leading to the Injury	"I was cleaning the pool, when I slipped on some leaves and fell into the deep end."

Shortly after initiating transport to the hospital, the patient experiences a marked decrease in sensation and movement in her lower extremities. Following reassessment of her vital signs, which remain stable, you advise your partner to divert to a trauma center. After starting an IV of normal saline, you contact medical control to advise them of the change in your patient's condition.

3. What medications are used to treat patients with spinal trauma?

_____

_____

_____

_____

A cardiac monitor is applied, which reveals a normal sinus rhythm at 80 beats/min. With an estimated time of arrival at the hospital of approximately 15 minutes, you perform an ongoing assessment **(Table 7-4)** and then call your report to the trauma center.

Table 7-4 Ongoing Assessment

Level of Consciousness	Conscious and alert to person, place, and time
Airway and Breathing	Airway remains patent; respirations, 18 breaths/min with adequate tidal volume
Oxygen Saturation	98% (on 100% oxygen)
Blood Pressure	120/80 mm Hg
Pulse	80 beats/min, strong and regular
ECG	Normal sinus rhythm

4. What type of shock is commonly associated with a spinal injury?

_____

_____

_____

_____

The patient is delivered to the trauma center and is immediately evaluated by the emergency department physician. A computer tomographic (CT) scan reveals a spinal cord contusion and swelling in the area of the sixth thoracic vertebrae. This is confirmed by a magnetic resonance imaging (MRI) scan.

The patient is admitted to the hospital. After 5 days of steroid therapy, neurologic function in her lower extremities improved. She fully recovered and was discharged home 2 days later.

1. What common mechanisms of injury cause spinal trauma?

Spinal injury should be suspected any time the patient has sustained a significant mechanism of injury (MOI) or when the MOI is unclear. The MOI plays a key role in assessing a patient and determining the most appropriate treatment. Specific MOIs that commonly cause spinal trauma include the following:

- **Flexion, extension, or hyperrotation**
  - These injuries can cause vertebral fractures and tearing of the ligaments and supporting musculature of the spinal column. The result is stretching of or impingement on the spinal cord, causing partial or complete spinal cord injury.
  - Flexion, extension, and rotation injuries often result from rapid deceleration mechanisms that are typically associated with motor-vehicle collisions. The spine is subjected to an abrupt forward motion as the vehicle rapidly decelerates (suddenly stops). The body is then secondarily propelled backward toward or beyond its original position **(Figure 7-1)**.

- **Lateral bending**
  - Because of the limited range of lateral motion of the spinal column, lateral bending injuries require less motion before spinal injury occurs. Following lateral impact (T-bone) of a car, the torso and thoracic spine move laterally. The head usually remains stationary until it is pulled to the side by the cervical attachments. This lateral movement results in damage to the cervical spinal ligaments and muscles as well as other supporting structures of the head.
    - Injuries secondary to excessive lateral movement of the spine include fractures and dislocations.

- **Axial loading**
  - Axial loading, or spinal compression, occurs when the forces of trauma are transmitted directly through the spinal column. This causes compression of the vertebra and can result in narrowing of the intervertebral spaces, shifting of the intervertebral discs, or fracturing of the vertebral bodies. Injuries caused by axial loading can result in impingement on the spinal cord, the spinal nerve roots or blood vessels, and partial or complete spinal cord injury.
  - Axial loading occurs when force is applied directly to the superior or inferior aspect of the spinal column. Patients can experience axial-loading injuries after jumping from a significant height (greater than three times the patient's height) and landing on their feet **(Figure 7-2)**, diving head first into shallow water, or striking a car's windshield with their head.

- **Distraction**
  - Distraction injuries occur when one part of the spine is stationary or stable and the other part is pulled in a longitudinal motion. This causes lacerations or tearing of the spinal ligaments, fractures of the vertebral discs, and stretching or tearing of the spinal cord (rarely). Hangings are classic examples of distraction injuries of the spine.
  - In some hanging injuries, the patient's weight causes a fracture of the second cervical vertebrae secondary to sudden hyperextension and distraction. This injury is commonly referred to as a "hangman's fracture."

- **Direct spinal trauma**
  - Direct trauma to the spinal column, as with your patient, can result in fractures of the spinal vertebrae and spinal cord compromise.

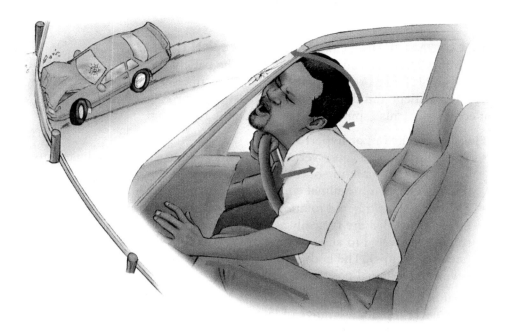

■ **Figure 7-1** Hyperextension injuries of the spine can occur when the patient's head strikes the windshield.

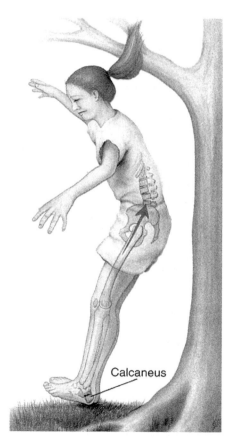

Calcaneus

■ **Figure 7-2** Axial-loading injuries of the spine can occur when a patient jumps from a significant height and lands on his or her feet.

Many significant spinal injuries are associated with high-speed motor-vehicle collisions, trauma above the level of the clavicles, and falls from greater than three times the patient's height. Direct trauma to the spinal column, though less common, can cause significant injury.

2. What are the specific types of spinal cord injury?

More than half of all spinal injuries involve the cervical spine. Thoracic injuries account for more than one-third of all spinal injuries, and lumbar and sacral injuries account for the remainder. Quadriplegia (paralysis of all four extremities) occurs secondary to injuries to the cervical spinal cord. Paraplegia (paralysis of the lower extremities) results from injuries to the thoracic or upper lumbar spinal cord.

Spinal cord injuries are classified as either primary or secondary. Primary injuries occur at the time of impact, and their effects are seen immediately. Primary injuries include concussions, contusions, compression injuries, lacerations, hemorrhagic injuries, and (rarely) transections **(Table 7-5)**.

Secondary injuries cause further damage to the cord after the initial insult and can be the result of swelling, ischemia, or the additional movement of unstable fractured vertebrae.

Table 7-5 Primary Spinal Cord Injuries

Concussion
- Occurs when the spinal cord moves within the spinal column, as with a cerebral concussion, which occurs when the brain moves around within the cranium.
- Spinal cord concussion usually results in temporary disruption of spinal cord function, and, in the absence of associated cord injury, typically does not cause permanent neurologic deficit.

Contusion
- Bruising of the spinal cord. This is typically associated with some tissue damage, bleeding, and swelling.
- Temporary disruption of spinal cord function distal to the site of the contusion is typically seen. However, unlike the concussion, the effects typically last longer, especially when significant swelling is involved. Contusions of the spinal cord often (but by no means always) resolve spontaneously with limited or no neurologic deficit.

Compression
- Compression injuries can occur secondary to displacement of fractured vertebrae, herniation of an intervertebral disc, or from swelling of adjacent tissue.
- Compression of the spinal cord results in compromise of cord circulation and ischemia and possibly physical damage to the cord. Neurologic deficits occur and, provided that the cord remains intact, may only be transient.

Laceration
- Lacerations can occur when bony vertebral fragments impinge on the spinal cord or if the cord is stretched to the point of tearing. Hemorrhage and swelling are likely to occur with this type of injury, causing loss of spinal cord function distal to the site of the injury.
- With minor lacerations, some recovery of neurologic function is possible; however, severe lacerations typically result in permanent neurologic deficit.

Hemorrhage
- Spinal cord hemorrhage is usually caused by contusions, lacerations, or stretching of the spinal cord.
- Pressure is placed on the cord due to the accumulation of blood in the area of the injury. Damage to the vasculature supplying the spinal cord and, therefore, neurologic function to distant parts of the body, may result in ischemia that extends above the level of the injury. Swelling causes temporary or permanent loss of cord function distal to the site of the injury.

Transection
- Transection (severing) of the spinal cord is very rare and can be caused by stretching or tearing of the cord or cord laceration caused by unstable fractured vertebrae.
  - Complete transection results in the loss of all sensory and motor functions distal to the injury.
  - Incomplete transection can be associated with preservation of some sensory and motor functions distal to the injury.

Transection of the spinal cord is almost always a primary injury; however, if unstable vertebral fragments move and impinge on the spinal cord after the initial injury, secondary transection can occur.

Most spinal cord injuries do not involve physical transection but instead are characterized by physiologic damage to the neurons. This results in functional transection that is broadly termed "spinal cord injury." Spinal cord injury can be categorized as partial or complete. With complete injuries, all spinal tracts are interrupted and all cord function distal to the area of the injury is lost. **Table 7-6** lists, by level of injury, the neurologic deficits associated with complete cord injury.

Table 7-6 Neurologic Deficit by Level of Spinal Injury

Above C3 (Brainstem)	Death secondary to complete loss of respiratory capability
C3 through C5	Quadriplegia and respiratory compromise
C6 through C8	Loss of arm movement and sensation
T1 through L2	Loss of trunk movement and sensation
Below L2	Paraplegia and incontinence

Complete spinal cord injury above the level of C3, in the region of the brainstem, typically results in death, because respiratory function is no longer possible. These patients often die before EMS arrives at the scene of the incident.

The phrenic nerves, which send motor impulses to the diaphragm, exit the spinal cord at C3, C4, and C5. A patient whose spinal cord is injured below the C5 level will lose the ability to move the intercostal muscles; however, because the phrenic nerves remain intact, diaphragmatic function will be preserved and the patient will be able to breathe spontaneously **(Figure 7-3)**.

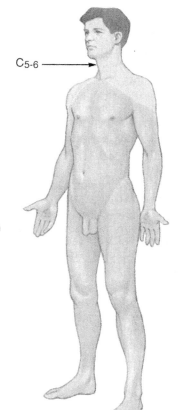

C5-6

Paralysis of
all muscles
below shoulders

Breathing by
diaphragm only

Loss of sensation
from shoulders down

■ **Figure 7-3** A patient whose spinal cord is injured below the level of C5 experiences quadriplegia; however, the patient can still breathe spontaneously because the phrenic nerves, which supply the diaphragm, originate at the C3, C4, and C5 levels.

With incomplete spinal cord injuries, some nerve tracts and motor–sensory functions remain intact. Although some degree of permanent neurologic deficit is likely, the prognosis for recovery is greater than with complete cord injuries. There are four specific types of incomplete cord injuries (Table 7-7), each of which causes varying types of neurologic deficit.

Table 7-7 Incomplete Spinal Cord Injury Syndromes

Anterior cord syndrome
- Often the result of hyperflexion injuries
- Occurs when bony vertebral fragments or pressure compress the arteries that supply the anterior cord. The cord is damaged by vascular disruption; its potential for recovery is poor.
- The patient will experience motor deficits with relative sensory sparing distal to the injury.
- Because only the anterior portion of the cord is affected, sensory response to light touch and proprioception (sense of position), which are functions of the posterior cord, are spared.

Central cord syndrome
- Often a result of contusion within the spinal cord
- Often occurs as the result of flexion or extension injury in individuals with increased susceptibility to injury secondary to developmental or degenerative narrowing of the spinal canal
- Because the central part of the cord contains nerve fibers that control the upper extremities, patients often present with sensory and motor deficits in the arms that are more severe than any deficits present in the legs.

Brown-Séquard's syndrome
- Less common type of incomplete spinal cord injury in which one half of the cord is affected
- Results in loss of sensory and motor functions on opposite sides of the body

Posterior cord syndrome
- Least common type of incomplete spinal cord injury
- Associated with loss of sensory function (typically pain, temperature, and vibration) with relative preservation of motor function distal to the zone of injury

3. What medications are used to treat patients with spinal trauma?

As previously discussed, the processes of swelling and inflammation can compound the initial physical injury to the spinal column or cord. Corticosteroids or steroids are commonly used to reduce the swelling, thereby relieving pressure on the spinal cord and facilitating recovery of neurologic function. Maximum benefits are seen if these drugs are administered within the first 8 hours after the injury. The following medications are commonly used in the emergency department setting:

■ **Methylprednisolone** (Solu-Medrol) is a synthetic glucocorticoid that possesses the potent anti-inflammatory properties of naturally occurring (endogenous) adrenal cortical steroids. High doses of methylprednisolone have been found to be effective in reducing the severity of spinal cord injury. The onset of action of methylprednisolone is 1 to 2 hours. The recommended dosing regimen is as follows:
- 30 mg/kg via IV push over 15 minutes within the first 8 hours after the injury
- After the initial bolus dose, an infusion at 5.4 mg/kg/hr is administered over the next 23 hours.
  - Methylprednisolone must be reconstituted prior to administration. It is supplied in a two-chamber vial (half powder and half liquid) and is reconstituted when the chambers are mixed.

■ **Dexamethasone** (Decadron, Hexadrol) is also a synthetic glucocorticoid that possesses anti-inflammatory effects. The onset of action of dexamethasone is 4 to 8 hours. The recommended dosing regimen following spinal cord injury is as follows:
- 4 to 24 mg via IV push as soon as possible after the injury
- Doses of up to 100 mg may be effective in some cases.

Because methylprednisolone has a faster onset of action than dexamethasone, it is usually the drug of first choice for spinal cord injury. You should understand local protocols related to the use of glucocorticoids in the prehospital setting. Because there is no demonstrated benefit of administration sooner than 6 to 8 hours following injury, and minimal demonstrated benefit compared with placebo overall, and because the potential long-term complications of high-dose glucocorticoid administration are devastating, steroids are very rarely administered in the field and are not even administered in the emergency department until after definite confirmation (by imaging and examination) of a specific spinal cord injury.

4. What type of shock is commonly associated with a spinal injury?

Neurogenic shock, also referred to as spinal shock, is the result of an interruption of sympathetic nervous system regulation of the body distal to the level of injury. Because sympathetic tone decreases, injury to the spinal cord results in dilation of the blood vessels distal to the site of injury.

Under normal circumstances (no spinal injury), baroreceptors, which are located throughout the body, sense decreases in blood pressure and send messages to the brain via the nervous system. The brain normally responds by sending messages to the sympathetic nervous system, which releases two catecholamines: epinephrine and norepinephrine. These catecholamines are responsible for vasoconstriction, which shunts blood from the periphery of the body to areas of greater need, as well as increased myocardial contractility (inotropy) and rate (chronotropy).

Loss of sympathetic tone causes vascular dilation with expansion of the vascular space, thus resulting in a "relative hypovolemia." In other words, relative to the now larger vascular space, blood volume is decreased, even though the patient has not actually lost any blood. Additionally, the lack of catecholamine release does not allow the body to compensate by increasing heart rate and contractility; therefore, stroke volume and cardiac output decrease and the patient experiences shock (hypoperfusion).

The patient in neurogenic shock typically does not present with the classic signs and symptoms that one would expect from other, non-spinal-injury-related shock (eg, hypovolemic, septic, anaphylactic). Signs of neurogenic shock include a normal or slow heart rate, hypotension, cool and moist skin above the level of the injury, warm and dry skin below the level of the injury, and priapism (sustained penile erection) in males.

Summary

Injury to the spine is a common occurrence associated with serious trauma and may result in significant disability or death. Some patients with significant spinal injury may present with minimal signs and symptoms; however, further manipulation of the spine may have disastrous consequences.

Signs and symptoms of spinal injury include pain in the area of injury and numbness or tingling in the extremities. More serious signs include deformity of the spinal column, paralysis, incontinence, priapism, and respiratory impairment.

Any patient with a significant mechanism of injury, such as high-speed motor-vehicle collisions, falls from greater than 20 feet (or three times the patient's height), or any serious trauma above the clavicles, should be assumed to have a spinal column injury until proven otherwise. Such patients must receive full spinal immobilization, oxygen as needed, careful transport to the hospital, and monitoring of neurologic function en route.

8

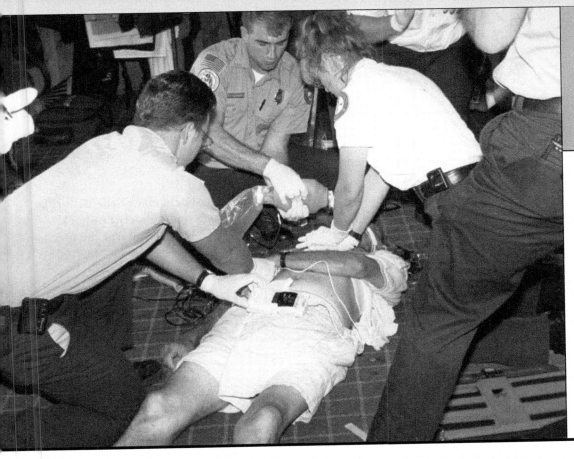

41-Year-Old Male with Traumatic Cardiac Arrest

At 9:55 PM, you are dispatched to 1344 West Bandera Avenue for a 41-year-old male with an unknown type of injury. While en route, the on-scene first responders advise you that CPR is in progress. You immediately notify dispatch and request a backup paramedic unit. Your response time to the scene is approximately 7 minutes.

1. What types of traumatic injuries commonly result in cardiac arrest?

You arrive at the scene at 10:02 PM. According to the patient's wife, her husband fell from an 8-foot ladder after being electrocuted while trimming tree branches near a high power line. First responders initiated CPR and delivered three shocks with the

AED prior to your arrival. After confirming pulselessness and apnea, you immediately attach a cardiac monitor and assess the patient's cardiac rhythm **(Figure 8-1)**.

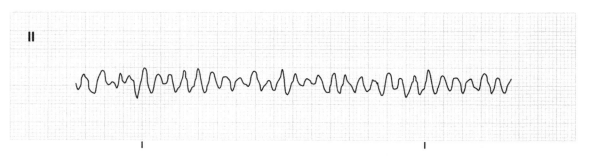

■ **Figure 8-1** Your patient's cardiac rhythm.

Recognizing the cardiac rhythm as being V-Fib, you immediately charge the defibrillator to 360 joules, ensure that all patient contact has ceased, and deliver the shock. The patient remains pulseless and apneic, so CPR is continued. Because of the mechanism of injury, the patient's spine is fully immobilized.

2. What is the pathophysiology of an electrical injury?

_____

_____

_____

_____

After 60 seconds of CPR, you glance at the cardiac monitor, which still reveals V-Fib. You deliver another defibrillation at 360 joules while your partner prepares the intubation equipment. In the meantime, the second paramedic unit arrives at the scene. With CPR ongoing, you perform a rapid trauma assessment of the patient **(Table 8-1)**.

Table 8-1 Rapid Trauma Assessment

Head	Contusion to the center of the forehead, no bleeding noted
Neck	Trachea is midline, jugular veins are flat, no cervical spine deformities.
Chest	Chest wall is symmetrical, no trauma noted, breath sounds are clear and equal bilaterally.
Abdomen/Pelvis	Abdomen is soft without bruising, pelvis is stable.
Lower Extremities	Closed deformity to left midshaft femur, apparent exit wound to bottom of left foot (covered with a sterile dressing)
Upper Extremities	Closed deformity to left midshaft humerus, apparent entrance wound to the palm of the left hand (covered with a sterile dressing)
Posterior	No deformities or bruising noted

The patient has been successfully intubated, and two large-bore IV lines of normal saline have been initiated. The patient is quickly loaded into the ambulance and transport to a local trauma center is begun. A paramedic from the second unit accompanies you in the back of the ambulance.

3. What pharmacological interventions are indicated for this patient?

_____

_____

_____

_____

The appropriate pharmacological interventions have been initiated and circulated with effective CPR. The patient remains in V-Fib, so you deliver another shock at 360 joules after 60 seconds. Following this shock, you assess the patient's cardiac rhythm, which has changed **(Figure 8-2)**.

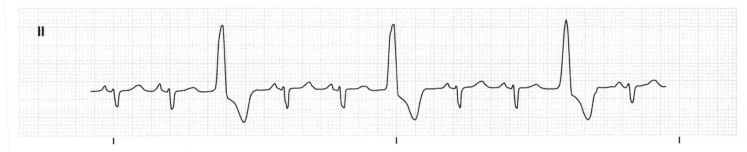

■ **Figure 8-2** Your patient's cardiac rhythm has changed.

The patient has a palpable carotid pulse that accompanies the new cardiac rhythm; however, his radial pulses are absent. He remains apneic and is being ventilated by your partner. Recognizing that the patient is significantly hypotensive, you prepare to administer IV fluids.

4. What are the goals of IV fluid therapy for this patient?

_____

_____

_____

_____

The appropriate IV fluid infusion has been initiated. With an estimated time of arrival at the hospital of 6 minutes, you perform an ongoing assessment of the patient **(Table 8-2)** and then call your radio report to the receiving facility. You then continue treatment to stabilize the patient's condition.

Table 8-2 Ongoing Assessment

Level of Consciousness	Unconscious and unresponsive
Airway and Breathing	Intubated and ventilated at 15 breaths/min
Oxygen Saturation	98% (ventilated with 100% oxygen)
Blood Pressure	94/56 mm Hg systolic
Pulse	94 beats/min and irregular, weak radial pulses
ECG	Sinus rhythm with ventricular trigeminy

5. What additional treatment is required for this patient?

_____

_____

_____

_____

You arrive at the emergency department and give your verbal report to the attending physician. The patient is placed on a mechanical ventilator, and radiographs of his deformed extremities are obtained. Blood chemistry analysis reveals electrolyte abnormalities and an arterial blood gas reveals metabolic acidosis. Following additional aggressive treatment in the hospital, the patient's condition stabilized. He later recovered and was transferred to a rehabilitation facility.

1. What types of traumatic injuries commonly result in cardiac arrest?

As with any patient in cardiac arrest, treatment must be directed at identifying and correcting the underlying cause, otherwise you will not be successful in your resuscitation efforts. Unfortunately, traumatic cardiac arrest secondary to blunt trauma has a very high mortality rate. This is because the injury leading to the arrest is typically disastrous. Such injuries include profound hypoxia, cervical spinal cord transection, and exsanguination (bleeding to death). However, unless the patient is exhibiting obvious signs of death (eg, rigor mortis, decapitation, burned beyond recognition), resuscitation should be attempted. **Table 8-3** lists the most common causes of cardiac arrest in the trauma patient.

Table 8-3 Causes of Cardiac Arrest in the Trauma Patient

Airway
- Foreign body obstruction (blood, broken teeth)
- Airway obstruction secondary to tongue prolapse
- Uncorrected hypoxia

Breathing
- Open pneumothorax (sucking chest wound)
- Tension pneumothorax
- Flail chest
- Paralysis of all muscles of respiration secondary to upper cervical spinal cord injury
- Carbon monoxide or cyanide toxicity
- Aspiration

Circulation
- Exsanguination
- Pericardial tamponade
- Massive myocardial contusion
- Electrocution

In addition to treating the cardiac arrest itself (ie, CPR, intubation, IV therapy), you must pay close attention to the mechanism of injury and carefully assess the patient in order to identify and immediately correct the underlying cause of the arrest. In some patients, you may discover more than one injury or condition that may have contributed to the cardiac arrest.

2. What is the pathophysiology of an electrical injury?

Electrical injuries account for approximately 6% of all burn center admissions and cause approximately 500 deaths each year. Males, construction workers, and golfers who fail to seek shelter during an electrical storm are at particularly high risk for electrical injury.

Your patient has experienced cardiac arrest secondary to a direct contact burn, which occurs when an electrical current directly penetrates the resistance of the skin and underlying tissues. To appreciate the damage caused by electrical injuries, a review of electrical current is in order.

The power of electricity is the result of electron flow from a point of high concentration to one of low concentration, much in the way that gases diffuse. The difference between the two electron concentrations is called voltage, which is the electrical potential between the two points. The rate of flow of an electrical charge is called the current and is measured in amperes, a measure of the strength of the electrical current.

Resistance, which is measured in ohms, is the degree of opposition offered by an object to the electrical current. Certain tissues of the body offer more resistance than others. For example, bone offers the greatest resistance to electrical current, whereas blood vessels and nerves offer the least resistance. Resistance is also affected by the presence or absence of a conductive medium, such as water. Wet skin, for example, decreases the resistance to electrical flow.

Electrical current can be high or low voltage and either direct current (DC) or alternating current (AC). Low-voltage direct current is less dangerous than low-voltage alternating current. This is because an alternating current follows the path of least resistance, which is usually the blood vessels and nerves, resulting in muscle tetany (ie, contractions), whereas direct current follows the shortest path.

Because an alternating current follows the path of least resistance, it can interfere with the control of muscle tissue. Current as low as 20 milliamperes (mA) can paralyze the diaphragm, causing respiratory arrest and death. As little as 50 mA can interfere with the cardiac electrical conduction system, causing ventricular fibrillation. Alternating current, commonly found in household currents, can cause tetany of the muscles with as little as 9 mA of current. Therefore, if a person comes in contact with a "live" wire, he or she may not be able to let go. This results in prolonged exposure to the electrical current, thereby increasing the severity of the injury.

Current that passes through large muscle masses may cause tetany severe enough to cause fractures and dislocations of the long bones (humerus and femur) as well as fractures and dislocations of the spinal vertebrae. Spinal injury can also occur due to falls following electrocution, as with your patient, who fell from a ladder.

Electrical injuries cause thermal burns because the resistance of the tissues converts the electrical current to heat. The amount of heat produced, and thus the severity of the electrical injury, is directly proportional to the type of current (AC or DC), strength of the current (amperage), resistance of the body's tissues, pathway of the current, and duration of contact **(Table 8-4)**. If any of these factors increase, the amount of heat produced, and thus the severity of the injury, will also increase. Small body parts that offer less resistance, such as the hands, fingers, toes, feet, and forearms, will sustain more damage than body parts that offer greater resistance, such as the trunk.

Table 8-4 Factors That Determine the Severity of an Electrical Injury

Type of voltage
Strength of the current
Resistance of the body's tissues
Pathway of the current
Duration of contact

Contact electrical burns produce an entrance and an exit wound. The hands and wrist are common entrance sites; the foot is a common exit site. The entrance wound, which typically resembles a bull's-eye, can be relatively small; however, do not let this deceive you. The degree of internal tissue damage can be and often is devastating **(Figure 8-3)**. The exit wound, like a large-caliber gunshot wound, is often extensive.

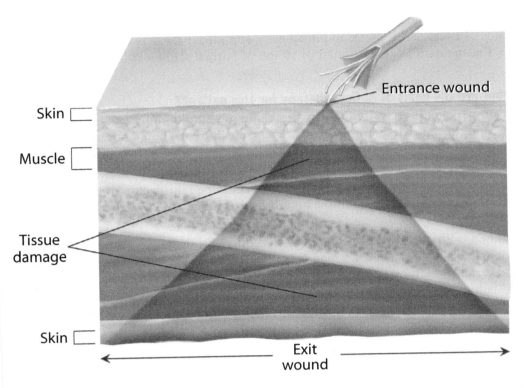

Skin

Muscle

Tissue
damage

Skin

Entrance wound

Exit
wound

■ **Figure 8-3** External signs of an electrical burn may be deceiving. The entrance wound may be a small burn, but damage to deeper tissue may be massive.

Muscles damaged by an electrical injury can undergo severe necrosis. Necrotic muscle releases myoglobin, a toxic chemical, into the blood stream, which can precipitate in the renal tubules and cause acute tubular necrosis, and therefore acute renal failure. Potassium is also released, which can cause severe hyperkalemia. Other organs may be damaged secondary to an electrical injury, including the abdominal organs and the bladder.

3. What pharmacological interventions are indicated for this patient?

The pharmacological interventions for a patient in V-Fib secondary to an electrical injury are the same as for the nontrauma patient. Defibrillation, of course, is clearly the most important intervention, and should be repeated every 60 seconds. Medications appropriate for this patient's condition include the following:

■ **Epinephrine 1 mg of a 1:10,000 solution**
  • Repeat every 3 to 5 minutes at the same dose.
  • There is no maximum dose for epinephrine in cardiac arrest.

Alternatively, you can administer vasopressin (Pitressin synthetic) in a one-time dose of 40 units via IV push in lieu of the *initial dose* of epinephrine. If vasopressin is administered, however, you should wait 10 to 20 minutes prior to administering epinephrine.

■ Administer **one** of the following antidysrhythmics:
  • **Lidocaine (Xylocaine) 1 to 1.5 mg/kg via IV push**
    • Repeat every 3 to 5 minutes
    • Maximum dose of 3 mg/kg
  • **Amiodarone (Cordarone) 300 mg via IV push**
    • Repeat at 150 mg 3 to 5 minutes later
    • Predilute in 20 to 30 mL of D_5W

Epinephrine and lidocaine can be administered via an endotracheal tube in the absence of IV access. If given endotracheally, administer these two drugs at 2 to 2.5 times the standard IV dose diluted in 10 mL of normal saline.

4. What are the goals of IV fluid therapy for this patient?

Your primary goal is to raise the patient's blood pressure to improve perfusion and prevent him from redeveloping cardiac arrest. Ideally, you should attempt to achieve a systolic blood pressure of 90 mm Hg, which is accomplished by administering 20 mL/kg fluid boluses of a crystalloid IV solution (eg, normal saline, lactated ringers).

Hypovolemia and hypotension in this patient could be multifactorial. It could be the result of the burn injuries, multiple long-bone fractures, or a low cardiac output state following cardiac arrest.

Additionally, the risk of renal complications is high following an electrical injury. As previously discussed, damaged muscles release myoglobin and potassium into the bloodstream, which can cause hyperkalemia, acute renal tubular necrosis, and acute renal failure. Therefore, crystalloid fluid infusions should be continued, even after achieving an acceptable blood pressure, to force diuresis and facilitate clearance of myoglobin and potassium from the bloodstream.

Although neither myoglobinuria nor urine output can be quantified in the prehospital setting, crystalloid fluids should be sufficient to maintain a urinary output of 75 to 100 mL/hr, which can be accomplished by infusing 500 mL of IV fluid per hour. Consult with medical control as needed regarding IV fluid infusions for patients with severe electrical injuries.

5. What additional treatment is required for this patient?

You have stabilized the patient's blood pressure with IV crystalloids; however, additional fluids will likely be required to ensure myoglobin clearance and adequate urinary output. You should consult medical control regarding additional fluid therapy.

The patient has a sinus rhythm with ventricular trigeminy (a PVC occurs every third beat), which indicates continued myocardial irritability. Therefore, an antidysrhythmic infusion is indicated. You should maintain a therapeutic blood level of the antidysrhythmic medication that aided in the successful resuscitation of the patient:

- Lidocaine
  - 1 to 4 mg/min, titrated to the desired effect
- Amiodarone
  - 360 mg IV over 6 hours (1 mg/min) followed by 540 mg IV over 18 hours (0.5 mg/min)
  - Maximum cumulative dose of 2.2 g in 24 hours

Sodium bicarbonate in a dose of 1 mEq/kg may be needed for this patient to treat hyperkalemia and metabolic acidosis, as well as to maintain an alkaline urinary output, further clearing myoglobin from the body. If sodium bicarbonate is administered, ensure that ventilations are delivered at the appropriate rate and depth. The use of digital capnometry can help quantify exhaled CO_2, allowing you to adjust ventilations accordingly. Sodium bicarbonate dissociates into carbonic acid (CO_2 and H_2O), which, in the absence of effective ventilation and oxygenation, can exacerbate intracellular acidosis.

Follow locally established protocols or contact medical control as needed regarding the administration of sodium bicarbonate during and after electrocution-induced cardiac arrest.

Patients with severe electrical injuries are also at risk for hypothermia; therefore, steps to maintain body temperature must be taken. Ensure that the heater is on in the back of the ambulance and place a blanket on the patient.

Summary

Electrical injuries result in a significant number of hospitalizations and are responsible for approximately 500 deaths each year. The vast majority of electrical injuries are caused by generated electricity, such as that encountered in power lines and household outlets.

It is important to understand the flow of electricity through the body and the negative effects that it has. Relative to the external damage caused by electrical injuries, internal damage is often more severe, and can include damage to nerves, blood vessels, and muscle. Damaged muscle releases myoglobin and potassium, which can precipitate in the kidneys and cause acute renal failure. Electrical current as low as 20 mA can cause respiratory arrest and as little as 50 mA can cause ventricular fibrillation.

Long-bone fractures and spinal injuries also can occur with severe electrical injuries and are caused by severe tetanic muscle spasms. Additionally, falls after being electrocuted are common. Therefore, the patient's spine must be immobilized to prevent further injury.

Contact electrical injuries, like gunshot wounds, typically produce an entrance and an exit wound. Compared to the entrance wound, the exit would is usually quite extensive. The hands and feet are common entry and exit sites.

Before treating the patient with an electrical injury, you must ensure that you, your partner, and any bystanders are safe. Do not touch the patient if the patient is still in contact with the electrical source and notify the power company as appropriate.

Patient care begins by ensuring airway patency, oxygenation, and ventilation. Administer 100% supplemental oxygen or assist ventilations as needed. Additional care involves spinal immobilization; covering burned areas with dry, sterile dressings; maintaining body temperature; administering crystalloid IV infusions to maintain adequate perfusion and to clear myoglobin from the urine; and rapidly transporting the patient to the appropriate facility. Consult with medical control as needed regarding the administration of sodium bicarbonate.

If the patient develops cardiac arrest, initiate CPR, defibrillate as needed, and administer medications in accordance with standard ACLS protocols.

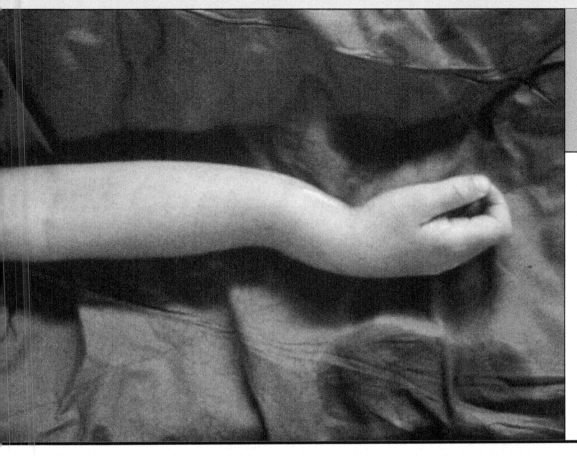

9

19-Year-Old Female with a Fractured Wrist

At 10:35 AM, you are dispatched to the parking lot of a local grocery store for a 19-year-old female with a possible broken arm. Your response time to the scene is less than 5 minutes.

You arrive at the scene at 10:39 AM, where you find the patient, who is conscious and alert, in considerable pain. A grocery store employee has applied ice to the injury site. While you perform an initial assessment of the patient (Table 9-1), your partner exposes the injury site, which reveals a closed deformity to the right wrist.

Table 9-1 Initial Assessment

Mechanism of Injury	Fell on outstretched hand
Level of Consciousness	Conscious and alert to person, place, and time
Chief Complaint	"I broke my arm. The pain is unbearable!"
Airway and Breathing	Airway is patent; respirations, normal rate and adequate tidal volume.
Circulation	Pulse, increased rate and strong; no bleeding is present; skin is pink, warm, and dry.

The patient denies other injuries and tells you that she felt a "snap" after falling on her outstretched right hand. She continues to complain of severe pain.

1. What complications are associated with fractures?

_____

_____

_____

While your partner maintains stabilization of the injured arm, you perform a focused physical examination (Table 9-2). The patient asks you to take her to the hospital because she cannot drive her car with the injured arm.

Table 9-2 Focused Physical Examination

Inspection	Deformity and swelling to the distal aspect of the wrist
Palpation	Skin distal to the injury site is pink, warm, and dry; pain and crepitus are noted upon palpation of the injury.
Distal Neurovascular Function	Radial pulse is present and strong, capillary refill time is less than 2 seconds, sensory and motor function are grossly intact.

2. What are the "six Ps" in evaluating an extremity injury?

_____

_____

_____

Following your focused assessment, the injury is splinted and the patient is placed into the ambulance. Prior to departing the scene, you obtain baseline vital signs and a SAMPLE history (Table 9-3).

Table 9-3 Baseline Vital Signs and SAMPLE History

Blood Pressure	106/68 mm Hg
Pulse	110 beats/min, strong and regular
Respirations	20 breaths/min, adequate tidal volume
Oxygen Saturation	98% (on room air)
Signs and Symptoms	Swollen, painful deformity to the right wrist; severe pain
Allergies	Erythromycin
Medications	None
Pertinent Past History	None
Last Oral Intake	Breakfast, 3 hours ago
Events Leading to the Injury	"I tripped and fell while carrying my groceries."

Transport is begun to a local hospital. The patient asks you if there is anything that you can do for her pain. You place an icepack over the injured area and elevate her arm.

3. What medications can be used to alleviate this patient's pain?

_____

_____

_____

You have administered the appropriate medication to the patient. While you are documenting this on your run report, the patient begins to complain that her right hand is tingling. You palpate her hand and note that it is cool. Additionally, her radial pulse is weaker than before.

4. What has likely happened? How will you remedy the situation?

_____

_____

_____

Following your intervention, the patient tells you that the tingling in her hand has resolved. Her radial pulse is strong and the extremity is warm. With an estimated time of arrival at the hospital of approximately 5 minutes, you perform an ongoing assessment **(Table 9-4)** and then call your report to the receiving facility.

Table 9-4 Ongoing Assessment

Level of Consciousness	Conscious and alert to person, place, and time
Airway and Breathing	Respirations, 16 breaths/min with adequate tidal volume
Oxygen Saturation	98% (on room air)
Blood Pressure	100/58 mm Hg
Pulse	80 beats/min, strong and regular

The patient is delivered to the hospital in stable condition. A radiograph is obtained, which confirms the presence of a Colles' fracture with an associated distal ulna fracture. After sedating the patient with midazolam (Versed) and injecting Lidocaine directly into the fracture site to provide pain relief, an orthopedic surgeon reduces the fracture (restores the radius to its normal alignment) and immobilizes it in a cast. Following observation for negative effects from the sedation, she is discharged from the emergency department and driven home by a friend.

1. What complications are associated with fractures?

Before discussing the complications associated with fractures, a brief discussion of this patient's injury is in order. Your patient has experienced a Colles' fracture, which is the most common fracture around the wrist. A Colles' fracture is characterized by a fracture and dorsal displacement of the radius. In many cases, the ulna also is fractured. The mechanism of injury most often associated with a Colles' fractures is a fall on an outstretched hand, resulting in dorsiflexion of the wrist. The associated deformity resembles a "dinner fork" **(Figure 9-1)**.

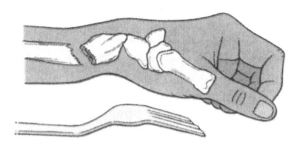

■ **Figure 9-1** The deformity associated with a Colles' fracture resembles a dinner fork.

Complications associated with fractures include hemorrhage, nerve damage, avascular necrosis, compartment syndrome, and fat embolism.

Because the skeleton is highly vascular, fractures may result in significant hemorrhage. This can be substantially worse if surrounding blood vessels, especially larger arteries and veins, are damaged. Although hemorrhage associated with a Colles' fracture is typically not life threatening, multiple long-bone fractures, bilateral femur fractures, or fractures of the pelvis can cause shock and death. **Table 9-5** lists the approximate internal blood loss associated with various fractures.

The ends of a fractured bone can impinge on adjacent nerves, causing partial or complete neurologic compromise distal to the fracture site. Complaints associated with nerve injury include distal parasthesias (pins and needles sensation), anesthesia (complete loss of sensation), paresis (weakness), or paralysis (loss of muscular control).

Avascular necrosis is another potential complication associated with fractures. When a bone is fractured, adjacent vascular damage can result in loss of flow of blood to portions of the bone itself. This results in ischemia of the bone marrow and eventual bone death.

Table 9-5 Internal Blood Loss Associated with Fractures

Humerus	500 to 750 mL
Radius or Ulna Shaft	250 to 500 mL
Hip	1,500 to 2,500 mL
Pelvis	1,000 to 4,000 mL
Femur	1,000 to 2,000 mL
Tibia or Fibula	500 to 1,000 mL

Compartment syndrome is caused by compromised perfusion due to increased pressure within an osteofascial compartment. Osteofascial compartments are formed when fascia, a tough and inelastic membranous connective tissue, connects with bone. These osteofascial compartments, which have minimal ability to expand, contain skeletal muscle, nerves, and vascular structures. Extremity fractures account for approximately 45% of all cases of compartment syndrome and typically involve closed fractures of the tibia, fibula, radius, femur, and distal humerus. Compartment syndrome can be associated with open or closed fractures.

When a bone is fractured, bleeding and edema may occur, causing pressure within the osteofascial compartment. If not treated, progressive swelling will compromise first venous return and then arterial inflow, ultimately resulting in tissue ischemia and necrosis. If pressure is not relieved (usually within 6 hours) following the injury, permanent damage will occur. In severe cases, the affected extremity may require amputation, especially if it is exposed to pressure for 8 hours or longer.

Compartment syndrome can have systemic effects as well. Damaged muscle releases myoglobin, a toxic chemical, as well as potassium, which can leak from the osteofascial compartment and cause electrolyte disturbances and renal complications.

Fat embolism is a common cause of secondary pulmonary injury following a fracture. Particles of fat may break free from a fracture site and travel as emboli to distant sites. The most common sites of secondary injury from these fat emboli are the lungs and the brain. Injury to the target organ (lung or brain) occurs as a result of toxic effects on the capillary membrane beds with a resultant increase in permeability resulting in pulmonary or cerebral edema.

2. What are the "six Ps" in evaluating an extremity injury?

Certain key elements should be included in your assessment of an injured extremity. These elements are aimed at identifying potential neurovascular compromise as well as the development of compartment syndrome. The "six Ps" **(Table 9-6)** mnemonic is a helpful tool when assessing a potentially fractured extremity.

Table 9-6 The Six Ps of Evaluating an Extremity Injury

Pain
- The patient typically complains of pain upon palpation or movement of the injured extremity.

Pallor
- Pallor distal to the injury site could indicate vascular compromise.
- Delayed capillary refill (>2 seconds) may also indicate vascular compromise.

Paralysis
- Difficulty or the inability to move an extremity is a common finding associated with a fracture.

Parasthesia
- Numbness or tingling distal to the injured site could indicate neurologic compromise.

Pressure
- The patient may complain of a feeling of tension within the injured extremity.
- Pressure indicates internal hemorrhage and swelling and could lead to compartment syndrome.

Pulselessness
- Diminished or absent distal pulses indicates vascular compromise.
- Distal pulses should be assessed before and after splinting and frequently thereafter.

If, when assessing a possible fractured extremity, you note that distal pulses are absent, gentle manipulation of the injury may be required to restore distal circulation. The decision to manipulate a possible fracture, however, should be based on your transport time to the hospital and at the discretion of medical control.

3. What medications can be used to alleviate this patient's pain?

Narcotic analgesics are frequently administered to patients in the prehospital setting to relieve pain associated with musculoskeletal injuries. The main therapeutic effects of these medications are that they decrease the patient's perception of pain and reduce anxiety. Commonly used narcotic analgesics include morphine sulfate, meperidine hydrochloride (Demerol), and nalbuphine hydrochloride (Nubain).

- **Morphine**
  - Administer in 2- to 4-mg increments via slow IV push.
    - May repeat every 2 to 3 minutes as needed
    - Prehospital dosing should not exceed 10 mg
- **Demerol**
  - Intramuscular (IM) injection
    - 50 to 100 mg from a prefilled syringe containing 100 mg/mL
  - IV administration
    - 50 to 100 mg from a single-dose vial containing 10 mg/mL
    - Dilute in a small volume of normal saline or lactated ringers
- **Nubain**
  - 10 mg/70 kg via IV, IM, or subcutaneous (SC) administration
  - May repeat at 2 mg as needed
  - Maximum single dose of 20 mg

Narcotic medications can depress the central nervous system and cause respiratory depression, hypotension, and bradycardia. Monitor the patient for these effects and be prepared to administer 0.4 to 2.0 mg of naloxone hydrochloride (Narcan) via IV or IM administration. Narcan is a narcotic antagonist that binds to opiate receptor sites in the body, thus reversing the deleterious effects of narcotics. Narcan, however, is a shorter-acting drug than most narcotics; therefore, repeat doses may be needed.

4. What has likely happened? How will you remedy the situation?

Although you cannot rule out the possibility of compartment syndrome, the splint has, in all likelihood, been applied too tightly. This is easily remedied by simply loosening the bandage securing the splint and resecuring it to achieve a looser fit. Do not, however, secure it so loosely as to defeat the purpose of the splint, which is to immobilize the injury. After resecuring the splint, reevaluate distal neurovascular status.

Pneumatic (air) splints are commonly used in the prehospital setting for immobilizing extremity injuries. Many paramedics and physicians do not favor air splints because they may actually facilitate the development of compartment syndrome. When using an air splint, inflate the device to the point where you can make a slight indentation in it with moderate finger pressure. If the patient complains of numbness or tingling, or if signs of vascular compromise are present (eg, weak distal pulse, cool extremity), simply release some of the air from the splint and reevaluate distal neurovascular function.

Summary

Unless associated with multiple systems trauma in which multiple long bones have been fractured, extremity injuries are rarely life threatening. However, if improperly managed, they may result in permanent disability.

Potential complications associated with fractures include hemorrhage, avascular necrosis, nerve damage, compartment syndrome, and fat embolism. Extremity injuries that have the greatest potential for severe blood loss include bilaterally fractured femurs, pelvic fractures, and multiple long-bone fractures.

Assessment of a potentially fractured extremity begins by manually stabilizing the extremity above and below the injury site. Assess distal neurovascular function by palpating for a distal pulse, assessing motor and sensory functions, feeling the temperature of the skin, and assessing capillary refill time.

Management includes splinting the extremity in the position found, unless neurovascular compromise is present. Depending on your transport time, medical control may order you to gently manipulate the injury to restore neurovascular function. After splinting the extremity, reassess distal neurovascular function.

If the patient complains of severe pain, narcotic analgesics may be administered. Such medications include morphine, Demerol, and Nubain. Follow locally established protocols or contact medical control as needed.

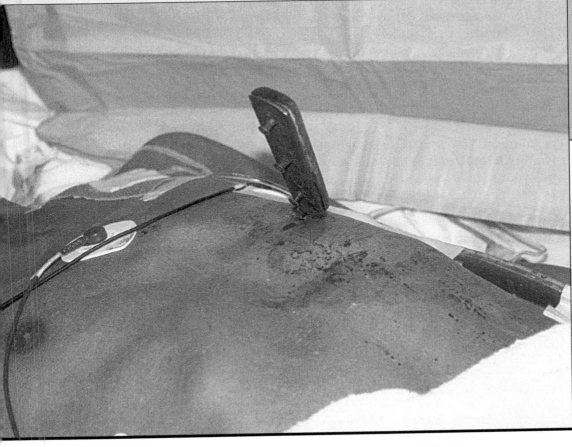

10

37-Year-Old Male with a Stab Wound

Law enforcement has requested your assistance at 344 West Kronkosky Street for an apparent stabbing that occurred during a domestic dispute. The scene is secure; the perpetrator, who is the patient's wife, has been apprehended. The time of the call is 1:20 AM, and your response time to the scene is approximately 6 minutes.

Upon arriving at the scene, you enter the residence, where you find the patient, a 37-year-old male with a large knife impaled in his anterior chest just below the left nipple. The patient is conscious, noticeably restless, and in obvious respiratory distress. You immediately perform an initial assessment of the patient **(Table 10-1)** while your partner opens the trauma bag.

1. What should you direct your partner to do while you assess the patient?

_____

_____

_____

_____

Table 10-1 Initial Assessment

Mechanism of Injury	Penetrating injury to the chest
Level of Consciousness	Conscious and alert, but restless
Chief Complaint	"I can't breathe!"
Airway and Breathing	Airway is patent; respirations, profoundly labored with reduced tidal volume.
Circulation	Radial pulses are rapid and weak; skin is cool, clammy, and pale; minimal bleeding from the site of the impaled knife; no other gross bleeding.

The injury site has been appropriately stabilized, and your partner has not discovered any other injuries or bleeding. You perform a rapid trauma assessment **(Table 10-2)** while your partner prepares to manage the patient's airway. A police officer quickly retrieves the stretcher from the ambulance.

2. How should you manage this patient's airway?

_____

_____

_____

_____

Table 10-2 Rapid Trauma Assessment

Head	No obvious trauma
Neck	Trachea is midline; jugular veins, flat; no cervical spine deformities.
Chest	Knife impaled in the anterior left chest, below the nipple (knife has been stabilized); breath sounds, markedly diminished on the left side of the chest; chest wall is dull to percussion on the left side.
Abdomen/Pelvis	Abdomen is soft and nontender, pelvis is stable.
Lower Extremities	No obvious trauma; pedal pulses, weakly present; sensory and motor functions, grossly intact
Upper Extremities	No obvious trauma; radial pulses, weakly present; sensory and motor functions, grossly intact
Posterior	No obvious trauma

After the appropriate airway management has been initiated, the patient is quickly loaded onto the stretcher and placed into the ambulance. After obtaining baseline vital signs and a SAMPLE history **(Table 10-3)**, you ask a police officer to drive the ambulance to the trauma center, because you need your partner's assistance in the back with the patient. After attaching a cardiac monitor and assessing the patient's cardiac rhythm **(Figure 10-1)**, you prepare to start two large-bore IV lines of normal saline.

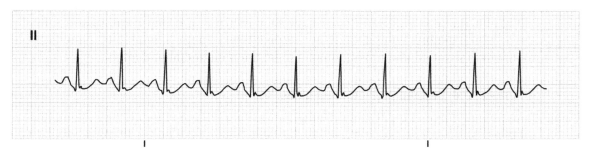

■ **Figure 10-1** Your patient's cardiac rhythm.

3. What type of intrathoracic injury is this patient experiencing?

_____

_____

_____

_____

Table 10-3 Baseline Vital Signs and SAMPLE History

Blood Pressure	88/58 mm Hg
Pulse	128 beats/min, weak and regular
Respirations	30 breaths/min, severely labored (ventilated with 100% oxygen)
Oxygen Saturation	93% (ventilated with 100% oxygen)
Signs and Symptoms	Signs of shock, knife impaled in anterior chest (stabilized)
Allergies	Unknown
Medications	Unknown
Pertinent Past History	Unknown
Last Oral Intake	Unknown
Events Leading to the Injury	According to law enforcement, "The patient's wife stabbed him during a domestic dispute."

4. How will you treat this patient's intrathoracic injury?

_____

_____

_____

_____

En route to the trauma center, your partner continues the appropriate airway management for the patient. The IV lines have been secured, and the appropriate fluid volume is being administered. With a transport time of approximately 15 minutes, you perform a detailed physical examination of the patient (Table 10-4).

Table 10-4 Detailed Physical Examination

Head	No obvious trauma to head or face; mouth and nose are clear; pupils equal and reactive to light.
Neck	Trachea is midline; jugular veins, flat; no cervical spine deformities.
Chest	Knife impaled in anterior chest (stabilized); breath sounds are diminished on left side; left side of chest is dull to percussion.
Abdomen/Pelvis	Abdomen is soft and nontender, pelvis is stable.
Lower Extremities	No obvious trauma; pedal pulses, weakly present; sensory and motor functions, grossly intact
Upper Extremities	No obvious trauma; radial pulses, weakly present; sensory and motor functions, grossly intact
Posterior	No obvious trauma

The patient remains conscious; however, he is still experiencing respiratory distress and is still restless. The appropriate airway management is continued and both IV lines remain patent and flowing. You reassess the stabilized knife in the patient's chest to ensure that it remains adequately secured.

5. Under which circumstances should you remove an impaled object?

_____

_____

_____

_____

Your estimated time of arrival at the hospital is 7 minutes. After performing an ongoing assessment of the patient (Table 10-5), you call your radio report to the receiving facility, where a trauma team is awaiting your arrival. The patient's condition appears to have improved somewhat.

Table 10-5 Ongoing Assessment

Level of Consciousness	Conscious, less restless
Airway and Breathing	Airway remains patent; respirations, 26 breaths/min (ventilated with 100% oxygen).
Oxygen Saturation	96% (ventilated with 100% oxygen)
Blood Pressure	94/50 mm Hg
Pulse	110 beats/min, stronger radial pulses
ECG	Sinus tachycardia

Upon arriving at the hospital, the trauma team greets you. After confirming a hemo-thorax on the left side of the chest, a 38-French chest tube is placed, which drains a significant amount of blood from the pleural space. The patient's blood pressure stabilizes, and he is taken to the operating room for removal of the knife and surgical repair of his injury. The patient recovered fully after a 10-day stay in the hospital.

10

1. What should you direct your partner to do while you assess the patient?

While you are assessing the patient's airway and breathing status, your partner should immediately stabilize the knife in the patient's chest. Obviously, the knife has not severed a major blood vessel (eg, aorta, vena cava) or directly penetrated the heart, otherwise the patient would be dead. Additionally, your partner should quickly assess the patient for other injuries that may require immediate bleeding control.

Though there are a variety of methods for stabilizing impaled objects, the goal is to prevent further injury by controlling external bleeding and preventing accidental movement of the impaled object. Slight movement on the proximal end of the impaled object can cause greater movement at the distal end. In the case of a knife impaled in the chest, this distal motion could easily lacerate large blood vessels, such as the aorta, vena cava, or coronary arteries, and cause exsanguination.

After controlling external bleeding from the injured site, the knife should be stabilized in place with bulky dressings, such as a trauma dressing or multiple gauze pads. Then, cover the knife with a protective barrier, such as a tall, rigid drinking cup or similar item **(Figure 10-2)**.

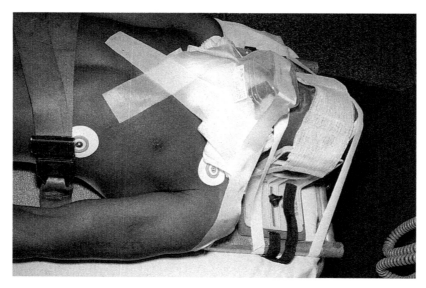

■ **Figure 10-2** After stabilizing the impaled object, tape a rigid item over the object to protect it from movement.

It is important that you and your partner communicate with each other, especially when managing a patient with a life-threatening injury. Treat the injuries that are going to be most rapidly fatal.

2. How should you manage this patient's airway?

Your patient's respirations, which are profoundly labored, are not producing adequate tidal volume. As a result, his minute volume will decrease as well, and he will develop respiratory arrest if you do not intervene immediately.

- Positive-pressure ventilatory support
  - Conscious patients are often resistant to assisted ventilations; however, failure to increase this patient's tidal volume (and minute volume) will result in worsened hypoxia.
  - Coach the patient and provide reassurance while you assist his ventilations with a BVM device and reservoir attached to 100% supplemental oxygen.

Ensuring adequate ventilation of a critically injured patient cannot be overemphasized. Passive oxygenation devices, such as a nonrebreathing mask, cannot provide positive pressure, and will be of little value to a patient with inadequate tidal volume.

Mechanical ventilation devices, such as the flow-restricted oxygen-powered ventilation device (FROPVD), deliver oxygen under high pressure (40 L/min) and should not be used to ventilate patients with thoracic trauma. High ventilatory pressures can cause or worsen barotrauma, resulting in exacerbation of the patient's condition.

If this patient's level of consciousness deteriorates, he will not be able to maintain his own airway and will have to be intubated.

3. What type of intrathoracic injury is this patient experiencing?

The assessment findings in this patient are highly suggestive of a hemothorax. In addition to the signs of shock (eg, diaphoresis, tachycardia, restlessness), the following clinical findings reinforce a field impression of hemothorax:

- **Decreased breath sounds** on the ipsilateral side as the injury, which indicates collapsing of the affected lung.
- **Labored breathing**, which indicates impaired ventilation secondary to collapsing of the lung.
- **Dullness to percussion**, also referred to as hyporesonance, is noted on the injured side and indicates blood within the pleural space. Air in the pleural space, as with a pneumothorax, produces a hyperresonant (high-pitched) note to percussion.
- **Flat jugular veins**, which is a later finding in a hemothorax, indicates significant hypovolemia.

A hemothorax occurs when blood collects in the pleural space and collapses the lung. Most often the result of a penetrating trauma, hemothorax is commonly accompanied by a pneumothorax (hemopneumothorax), in which case both air and blood accumulate in the pleural space **(Figure 10-3)**. Blood and/or air in the pleural space cause progressive collapsing of the lung, impaired ventilation, and hypoxia.

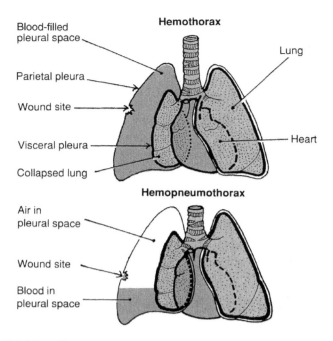

Figure 10-3 (A.) A hemothorax occurs when blood accumulates in the pleural space. (B.) A hemopneumothorax occurs when a combination of blood and air accumulate in the pleural space.

In the adult, each hemithorax (half of the chest) can accommodate approximately 3,000 mL of blood, which is half of the total blood volume. However, severe hemodynamic compromise typically occurs when 1,000 mL of blood or more accumulates in the pleural space.

Hemorrhage within the pleural space can come from different sources. Most commonly, the source of bleeding is damage to the parenchyma (tissue) of the lung. Other structures that can sustain damage from penetrating trauma include the intercostal vasculature and the great vessels (ie, vena cava, aorta). Blunt trauma, though less common, also can cause a hemothorax. Small hemothoraces, caused by minor internal bleeding, may not be detected in the field.

Approximately 25% of patients with severe thoracic trauma experience a hemothorax. Massive hemothoraces have a mortality rate of approximately 75%, with nearly two-thirds of these patients dying at the scene of the injury.

The signs and symptoms of a hemothorax, which are summarized in **Table 10-6**, are representative of hypovolemic shock and respiratory compromise. The clinical presentation is typically that of shock (eg, restlessness, tachycardia, hypotension), diminished or absent breath sounds on the ipsilateral side, dull percussion on the affected side, and varying degrees of respiratory distress.

With a hemopneumothorax, hyperresonance (a high-pitched note) may be noted upon percussion of the apices of the lungs, with hyporesonance noted at the bases. This is because air has a tendency to rise and blood has a tendency to settle. The external jugular veins may be normal, especially if the hemothorax is small. Massive hemothoraces, however, are associated with severe hypovolemia and typically result in collapsed jugular veins. The trachea is typically found in a midline position; however, in cases of massive hemothorax, contralateral deviation of the trachea may be noted.

Table 10-6 Signs and Symptoms of Hemothorax

Signs of shock
Respiratory distress
Diminished or absent breath sounds on the ipsilateral side
Dull (hyporesonant) percussion on the ipsilateral side
Normal or flat jugular veins
Contralateral tracheal deviation (late)

The prehospital environment can be a loud, uncontrolled setting. Therefore, it may be difficult to differentiate between a hemothorax, tension pneumothorax, and pericardial tamponade, especially if the patient is extremely restless. **Table 10-7** lists the clinical findings associated with each of these three conditions.

Table 10-7 Differential Diagnosis of Severe Chest Trauma

Assessment	Hemothorax	Tension Pneumothorax	Pericardial Tamponade
Pulse	Rapid	Rapid	Rapid
Blood pressure	Low or normal	Low	Low
Breath sounds	Diminished or absent	Absent	Bilaterally equal
Jugular veins	Normal or flat	Distended	Distended
Percussion	Dull	Hyperresonant	Normal
Trachea	Midline or deviated	Deviated (late)	Midline

4. How will you treat this patient's intrathoracic injury?

Initial management of a hemothorax, as with any critical injury, includes ensuring adequate ventilation and oxygenation. Your partner is already addressing this patient's inadequate breathing with positive-pressure ventilatory support and 100% oxygen.

After initiating two large-bore IV lines, infuse isotonic crystalloid fluids to maintain adequate perfusion (eg, improved mental status). Ideally, you should maintain a systolic blood pressure of 90 mm Hg. The goal is to maintain the systolic blood pressure, not increase it. Caution must be exercised when administering IV fluid boluses to the patient with intrathoracic hemorrhage. Rapid fluid infusions can cause a sudden increase in the systolic blood pressure and exacerbate internal bleeding. Follow locally established protocols or contact medical control regarding IV fluid resuscitation for a hemothorax.

Continuous cardiac monitoring of the patient with an intrathoracic injury is essential. Intrathoracic pressure can compress the myocardium, resulting in life-threatening cardiac dysrhythmias. Additionally, cardiac arrest may develop and is often associated with pulseless electrical activity (PEA).

If a hemopneumothorax is suspected, as evidenced by absent breath sounds on the ipsilateral side and hyperresonant percussive sounds over the apex of the affected lung, medical control may order you to perform a needle thoracentesis, also referred to as a chest decompression. Removing air from the pleural space in a hemopneumothorax may allow for partial reexpansion of the affected lung and improve the patient's condition until the injury can be repaired surgically. Clearly, partial improvement is better than no improvement, especially if the patient is hemodynamically unstable. Needle thoracentesis, however, is of no value if there are no signs of air in the pleural space (eg, massive hemothorax).

Needle thoracentesis is performed by inserting a large-bore (14-gauge) IV catheter into the second intercostal space in the midclavicular line. Intercostal nerves, arteries, and veins lie on the inferior border of each rib; therefore, you must follow the superior border of the third rib when inserting the IV catheter into the pleural space. As with a tension pneumothorax, contralateral tracheal deviation is a late sign of a tension hemopneumothorax; therefore, you must not wait for this sign to appear before performing needle thoracentesis. Following needle thoracentesis, whether air is removed from the pleural space or not, the IV catheter should be secured in place.

Delays must not occur in the field with the patient experiencing a hemothorax, because definitive care cannot be achieved in the prehospital setting. Immediate care in the emergency department involves performing a tube thoracostomy (placing a chest tube) to remove blood from the pleural space, allowing reexpansion of the collapsed lung. A tube thoracostomy is performed by inserting a large-bore (38-French or larger) chest tube into the fourth intercostal space in the midaxillary line. Many times, simply draining the hemothorax and allowing bleeding to spontaneously stop is all that is necessary. If bleeding is excessive and ongoing, definitive care is provided by surgical intervention.

Prehospital care for a hemothorax should focus on ensuring adequate oxygenation and ventilation, maintaining adequate perfusion with IV crystalloid fluids, and rapidly transporting the patient to a trauma center.

5. Under which circumstances should you remove an impaled object?

In the vast majority of circumstances, impaled objects should not be removed. Doing so will cause further damage to tissue and vasculature, perhaps worse than the damage caused by the initial injury. Stabilize the impaled object where and as it is found and transport the patient promptly.

However, select circumstances may require the removal of an impaled object from the patient. If the object is impaled in the airway or is otherwise making airway management impossible, it should be carefully removed. An example of this is an object impaled through the cheek and causing airway compromise. In this case, the object should be removed in the same direction that it entered, and any oral bleeding controlled.

Impaled objects should also be removed if they interfere with your ability to perform CPR. An example of this would be a knife or other object impaled in the precordium in a patient in cardiac arrest, which would directly interfere with chest compressions, or an object impaled in the back in a patient in cardiac arrest, making it impossible to place the patient in a supine position. In such cases, carefully remove the object, control external bleeding, perform CPR, and rapidly transport the patient to the trauma center.

Summary

Hemothorax can be fatal in patients with penetrating chest trauma. A person can lose his or her entire blood volume into the chest cavity, because each hemithorax can accommodate 3,000 mL of blood. As blood leaves the intravascular compartment and fills the pleural space, the patient develops hypovolemic shock. Additionally, blood in the pleural space causes progressive collapse of the affected lung, compromising ventilation and oxygenation.

Suspect a hemothorax with any case of penetrating trauma to the chest. The patient is likely to present with shock, diminished or absent breath sounds on the affected side, hyporesonance to percussion on the affected side, and, in severe cases of hypovolemia, collapsed jugular veins.

Pneumothorax accompanies many hemothoraces, which can make it difficult to differentiate hemothorax from a pneumothorax. If hemopneumothorax is suspected and severe respiratory distress with shock is present, medical control may order you to perform a needle thoracentesis to remove air from the pleural space to allow for at least partial reexpansion of the collapsed lung. Doing so may improve the patient's condition.

Impaled objects should not be removed in the prehospital setting unless they compromise the airway or interfere with your ability to perform CPR. Stabilize impaled objects where and as they are found with bulky dressing and then place a rigid barrier over the object to protect it from movement.

Prehospital management for a hemothorax includes ensuring effective ventilation and oxygenation, maintaining adequate perfusion with IV crystalloid fluids, and rapidly transporting the patient to a trauma center for the placement of a chest tube and further evaluation of the injury.

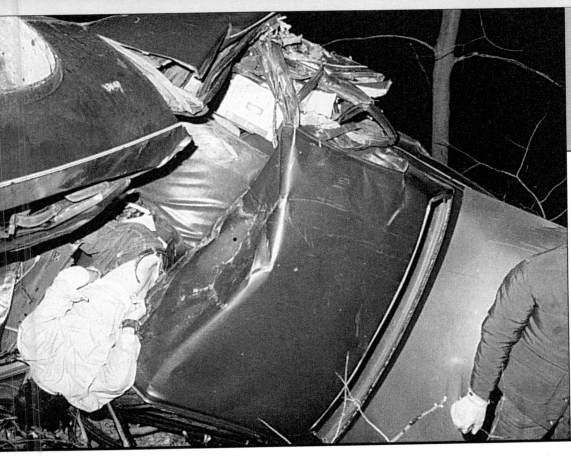

11

31-Year-Old Female's Passenger is Killed in a Car Crash

At 11:37 PM, you are dispatched to the scene of a motor-vehicle crash that is approximately 8 miles outside the city limits on Highway 46. Law enforcement personnel, who are already at the scene, notify you that a fatality is involved. The fire department is also en route to the scene.

Upon arriving at the scene, you size up the situation. The first patient, a young male, was partially ejected from the vehicle when it rolled over multiple times and is now deceased. The second patient is a 31-year-old female who is sitting on the ground holding her arm. She tells you that she was wearing her seatbelt, but her boyfriend was not. The fire department arrives at the scene shortly after your arrival.

1. What mechanisms of injury warrant transport of the adult patient to a trauma center in the absence of other evidence of significant injury?

_____

_____

_____

_____

Your partner immediately manually stabilizes the patient's head while you perform an initial assessment **(Table 11-1)**. The patient, who is crying, tells you that her left arm hurts. She denies a loss of consciousness before or after the accident.

Table 11-1 Initial Assessment

Mechanism of Injury	Rollover motor-vehicle crash, fatality in the same vehicle
Level of Consciousness	Conscious and alert to person, place, and time
Chief Complaint	Left arm pain
Airway and Breathing	Airway is patent; respirations, slightly increased with adequate tidal volume.
Circulation	Radial pulse is increased, strong, and regular; minor bleeding from abrasions to the forehead and a laceration to the left arm; skin is pink, warm, and dry.

2. What injuries should you anticipate based on the mechanism of injury?

_____

_____

_____

_____

Your partner maintains manual stabilization of the patient's head. You attempt to apply supplemental oxygen to the patient; however, she tells you that she does not need it. On the basis of the mechanism of injury, you perform a rapid trauma assessment of the patient **(Table 11-2)**. A firefighter retrieves the spinal immobilization equipment from the ambulance.

Table 11-2 Rapid Trauma Assessment

Head	Abrasion to the center of the forehead, no other trauma noted
Neck	Trachea is midline; jugular veins, normal; no cervical spine deformities.
Chest	Chest movement is symmetrical; no bruising or deformities noted; breath sounds are clear and equal bilaterally to auscultation.
Abdomen/Pelvis	Abdomen is soft and nontender; pelvis is stable.
Lower Extremities	No obvious trauma; pedal pulses, present and equal; sensory and motor functions, grossly intact
Upper Extremities	One-inch laceration to the left forearm; radial pulses, present and equal; sensory and motor functions, grossly intact
Posterior	No obvious trauma

The patient is apprehensive about being transported to the hospital; however, after explaining the potential seriousness of the situation, she agrees to EMS transport. The patient's spine is fully immobilized, and she is placed into the ambulance. You obtain baseline vital signs and a SAMPLE history **(Table 11-3)** and then depart the scene.

Table 11-3 Baseline Vital Signs and SAMPLE History

Blood Pressure	122/82 mm Hg
Pulse	110 beats/min, strong and regular
Respirations	20 breaths/min, adequate tidal volume
Oxygen Saturation	98% (on room air)
Signs and Symptoms	One-inch laceration to the left forearm, abrasion to the center of the forehead
Allergies	No drug allergies
Medications	None
Pertinent Past History	None
Last Oral Intake	Supper, 3 hours ago
Events Leading to the Injury	"I lost control of the car when I rounded a corner too fast."

3. What treatment should you provide to this patient?

_____

_____

_____

_____

While en route to the hospital, you dress and bandage the laceration on the patient's forearm and then perform a detailed physical examination **(Table 11-4)**. Your estimated time of arrival at the hospital is 12 minutes.

Table 11-4 Detailed Physical Examination

Head and Face	Abrasion to the center of the forehead; nose and mouth are clear; no deformities to the skull; pupils are equal and reactive to light.
Neck	Trachea is midline; jugular veins are normal.
Chest	Chest movement is symmetrical; no bruising or deformities noted; breath sounds are clear and equal bilaterally to auscultation.
Abdomen/Pelvis	Abdomen is soft and nontender; pelvis is stable.
Lower Extremities	No obvious trauma; pedal pulses, present and equal; sensory and motor functions, grossly intact
Upper Extremities	Laceration to the left forearm (bandaged); radial pulses, present and equal; sensory and motor functions, grossly intact
Posterior	Evaluated during rapid trauma assessment; patient is fully immobilized.

Supplemental oxygen is again offered to the patient; however, she still refuses to accept it. The patient also tells you that she does not want an IV. You continue to monitor the patient for signs of internal bleeding and shock.

4. How can you estimate the severity of blood loss in a patient?

_____

_____

_____

_____

The patient's condition remains stable throughout transport. With an estimated time of arrival at the hospital of 5 minutes, you perform an ongoing assessment **(Table 11-5)** and then call your report to the receiving facility.

Table 11-5 Ongoing Assessment

Level of Consciousness	Conscious and alert to person, place, and time
Airway and Breathing	Airway remains patent; respirations, 18 breaths/min; adequate tidal volume
Oxygen Saturation	98% (on room air)
Blood Pressure	118/80 mm Hg
Pulse	94 beats/min, strong and regular

Upon arriving at the trauma center, an emergency physician immediately evaluates the patient. Physical examination and radiographic evaluations reveal no life-threatening injuries. Following suturing of the laceration to her arm, the patient is discharged.

1. What mechanisms of injury warrant transport of the adult patient to a trauma center in the absence of other evidence of significant injury?

A crucial component of the scene size-up is careful assessment of the mechanism of injury (MOI). Many times, this may serve as your only indicator of a patient's need for transport to a trauma center. Your index of suspicion of potential injuries will be based on the information obtained from evaluating the MOI.

The decision to transport a patient to a trauma center versus the nearest hospital can be a difficult one. This is especially true if the MOI is unclear and if the patient does not present with significant signs and symptoms suggestive of life-threatening injuries. However, it is always better to err on the side of caution and immediately transport such patients to a trauma center.

Predefined trauma triage criteria are used to determine a patient's need for transport to a trauma center versus a local hospital. The criteria listed in **Table 11-6** apply to the adult patient and are especially helpful when the patient does not appear to be critically injured. Remember, trauma patients may present with very subtle signs and symptoms initially, only to rapidly deteriorate later.

Many patients who are transported to a trauma center on the basis of the MOI do not have life-threatening injuries; however, this is a determination that must be made by a physician at a trauma center, not by the paramedic in the field.

Table 11-6 Trauma Triage Criteria for Direct Transport to a Trauma Center

Significant falls
• Falls greater than 20 feet
• Falls more than three times the patient's height
Ejection from a motor vehicle
Rollover of a motor vehicle
Pedestrian/bicyclist struck by motor vehicle
• Struck by a vehicle traveling greater than 5 MPH
• Thrown or run over by a vehicle
Motorcycle impact greater than 20 MPH
Severe vehicular impact
• Impact speed greater than 40 MPH
• Vehicle deformity greater than 20 inches
• Occupant compartment intrusion of greater than 12 inches
Death of another occupant in the same vehicle
Extrication time of greater than 20 minutes

2. What injuries should you anticipate based on the mechanism of injury?

Your patient has been exposed to multiple, significant mechanisms of injury. These include rollover of a vehicle, severe vehicular impact, and death of an occupant in the same vehicle. Although the patient does not appear to be critically injured, you must assume that she experienced the same forces that killed the passenger.

During a vehicle rollover, the patient, the patient's internal organs, and the vehicle may sustain multiple impacts at different angles; therefore, the injury patterns are unpredictable, and the potential for severe injuries is significant. The severity of injuries sustained during a vehicle rollover is magnified if the patient is ejected from the vehicle. The mortality rate following a rollover crash is significantly higher if the patient is ejected from the vehicle.

Injury patterns following a rollover crash are most unpredictable when the victim is unrestrained. This is because the unrestrained patient usually strikes the interior of the vehicle multiple times.

Even when restrained, such as with your patient, passengers can sustain severe injuries during a rollover crash. However, the injury patterns tend to be more predictable and the injuries less severe. The passenger on the outboard side of the vehicle is at highest risk for injury, because the passenger is typically pinned against the door. This can cause injuries to the lateral aspect of the body, including lateral bending of the neck and lateral chest and pelvic injuries.

Because of the significant forces created during a rollover crash, restrained occupants may sustain shearing-type injuries, as seen with rapid-deceleration motor-vehicle crashes. Although the occupant is held secure by the restraint system, the internal organs can still move and can be injured as a result. Shearing-type injuries can involve the great vessels (ie, aorta, vena cava), tearing of the ligamentum arteriosum (supporting structure of the aorta), and tearing of the ligamentum teres (the supporting structure of the liver). These injuries typically result in death due to massive internal hemorrhage.

When the roof of the vehicle strikes the ground, the restrained occupant can still move toward the roof, impacting it with the head. This can cause axial-loading injuries to the cervical spine. Rollover crashes are particularly dangerous for both restrained and, to a greater degree, unrestrained occupants, because they provide multiple opportunities for second and third collisions.

3. What treatment should you provide to this patient?

You are already rendering the most important treatment for this patient, which is transporting her to a trauma center for evaluation. Although your assessment has not revealed any external life-threatening injuries, the patient could be experiencing slow internal bleeding, in which case the signs and symptoms may not yet be evident. The tachycardia that the patient is experiencing could be the result of emotional upset; however, you should interpret it as a possible sign of shock. Treatment for this patient, most of which you have already provided, is as follows:

■ Spinal immobilization
  • The mechanism of injury clearly suggests the potential for spinal injury.
  • Do not let the absence of pain or obvious spinal injury deter you from providing spinal immobilization.

■ 100% supplemental oxygen
  • Although the patient has refused oxygen, a nonrebreathing mask set at 15 L/min would be appropriate.
  • You should explain to the patient that her tachycardia could indicate internal bleeding and that oxygen is needed.

■ IV therapy
  • If local protocol requires you to start an IV on patients who are transported to a trauma center on the basis of the MOI, start at least one large-bore IV with normal saline or lactated ringers and set the flow rate to keep the vein open.
  • Be aware that the uninjured patient may refuse IV therapy.

■ Transport to a trauma center
  • As previously discussed, the mechanisms of injury associated with this motor-vehicle crash should increase your index of suspicion for serious injuries.
  • Any patient who experiences a significant mechanism of injury deserves evaluation in a trauma center, regardless of his or her initial clinical presentation.

The patient may think that your treatment is unnecessary because she feels fine. You should explain that due to the severity of the motor-vehicle crash, the potential for serious injury exists, and that even though she feels fine now, she could deteriorate later. Ensure that the patient understands the rationale for your actions and that they are in her best interest.

4. How can you estimate the severity of blood loss in a patient?

As previously discussed, this patient may have sustained internal injury and not yet developed signs and symptoms. Because of the mechanism of injury (rollover), this patient may have experienced the shearing forces previously discussed, which can cause internal hemorrhage from small lacerations of the liver, spleen, or other organs. You must monitor this patient carefully for early signs of shock. The severity of internal blood loss can only be estimated by performing careful, systematic, and frequent assessments of the patient.

Healthy adults (assumed to weigh 70 kg) can tolerate blood loss of up to 750 mL, or 15 percent of their total blood volume. This amount of bleeding, which is similar to donating approximately one unit of blood, is easily tolerated by the normal, healthy adult. Therefore, the patient may only experience slight anxiety and a widening pulse pressure, or, the patient may be completely asymptomatic. Frequent assessment of the patient is the only way that you will detect subtle vital sign changes.

Just as a "normal" blood pressure varies from person to person, so does the blood pressure required to maintain adequate perfusion. Furthermore, the body's systems compensate to maintain arterial blood pressure (eg, tachycardia, vasoconstriction). However, most texts and clinicians agree that a systolic blood pressure of less than 90 mm Hg in the adult trauma patient is clinically significant.

Although the patient's blood pressure should be monitored frequently to detect changes, more reliable assessment tools are available to identify the early signs of shock in the trauma patient. These include mental status, pulse rate and quality, respiratory rate and quality, and skin condition and temperature. Hypotension may not occur until the patient has lost 30 percent of his or her total blood volume or more.

According to the American College of Surgeons, there are four classifications of hemorrhage, each of which affects the patient's vital signs differently (Table 11-7). This classification system assumes a healthy adult patient who weighs 70 kg.

Table 11-7 Classifications of Hemorrhage

Class I Hemorrhage
- Less than 15 percent (750 mL) blood volume loss
  - Mental status: normal or slight anxiety
  - Pulse rate: less than 100 beats/min
  - Pulse pressure: normal or widened
  - Respiratory rate: 12 to 20 breaths/min
  - Blood pressure: normal

Class II Hemorrhage
- 15 to 30 percent (750 to 1,500 mL) blood volume loss
  - Mental status: mild anxiety
  - Pulse rate: greater than 100 beats/min
  - Pulse pressure: narrowed
  - Respiratory rate: 20 to 30 breaths/min
  - Blood pressure: normal

Class III Hemorrhage
- 30 to 40 percent (1,500 to 2,000 mL) blood volume loss
  - Mental status: confusion and anxiety
  - Pulse rate: greater than 120 beats/min
  - Pulse pressure: narrowed
  - Respiratory rate: 30 to 40 breaths/min
  - Blood pressure: decreased

Class IV Hemorrhage
- Greater than 40 percent (2,000 mL) blood volume loss
  - Mental status: lethargy or unconsciousness
  - Pulse: greater than 140 beats/min
  - Pulse pressure: narrowed
  - Respiratory rate: greater than 35 breaths/min
  - Blood pressure: markedly decreased or unobtainable

Summary

Assessing the mechanism of injury is a critical component in the overall evaluation of a trauma patient. Although the patient may present with relatively stable vital signs and no obvious trauma, a careful assessment is crucial in order to identify early signs of internal hemorrhage and shock.

The paramedic should maintain a high index of suspicion when assessing the patient involved in an incident associated with a significant mechanism of injury. Such incidents include, among others, falls from greater than 20 feet, death of an occupant in the same car following a motor-vehicle collision, and major vehicular damage.

Motor-vehicle collisions, especially rollovers, can cause a variety of life-threatening injuries; however, serious signs and symptoms may not be immediately evident following the injury. The patient may be stable initially; however, if the mechanism of injury suggests the potential for life-threatening injuries, the paramedic should treat the patient accordingly and transport the patient to a trauma center.

Many patients, who, based solely on the mechanism of injury, are transported to a trauma center, do not have significant trauma. Other patients, however, who are asymptomatic at the scene and refuse transport following a significant mechanism of injury, later deteriorate or die as the result of internal injuries, because the signs and symptoms of the injuries were not immediately evident.

In the best interest of the patient, the paramedic should transport anyone with a significant mechanism of injury to a trauma center, regardless of his or her clinical presentation.

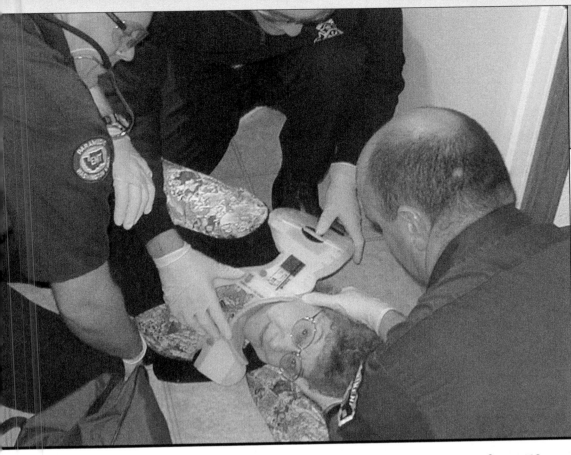

12

70-Year-Old Female with a Hip Fracture

At 9:20 AM, you are dispatched to 517 West Graham Street for a 70-year-old female who has fallen. The patient's neighbor, who checks in on her from time to time, discovered the woman after she did not answer her phone. Your response time to the scene is approximately 10 minutes.

You arrive at the scene at 9:30 AM. Upon entering the residence, you find the patient lying on her left side in her living room. She tells you that she fell the prior day, but cannot remember the exact time. Your partner provides manual inline stabilization of the patient's head while you perform an initial assessment (Table 12-1).

Table 12-1 Initial Assessment

Mechanism of Injury	Fall
Level of Consciousness	Conscious, but confused
Chief Complaint	"My left hip hurts."
Airway and Breathing	Airway is patent; respirations, normal rate and quality.
Circulation	Radial pulse, normal rate and regular; no gross bleeding

1. What are common contributing factors to falls in the elderly?

_____

_____

_____

Because of her confusion, you place the patient on supplemental oxygen. You perform a focused physical examination **(Table 12-2)** while your partner maintains manual stabilization of the patient's head. The neighbor goes into the kitchen to retrieve the patient's medications.

Table 12-2 Focused Physical Examination

Inspection	Lateral rotation of the left foot, left leg appears shorter than the right
Palpation	Pain to left hip upon palpation and with movement of the left leg; no crepitus noted
Neurovascular	Pedal pulses are present bilaterally; gross sensory and motor functions appear intact bilaterally.
Time of Injury	"Yesterday, but I cannot remember the exact time."

Further examination of the patient reveals the presence of severe kyphosis. Because of the mechanism of injury, you apply a cervical collar and prepare to immobilize the patient's spine. According to the neighbor, the patient is usually well oriented and not confused.

2. What are some common causes of altered mental status in the elderly?

_____

_____

_____

3. What is kyphosis? How will you immobilize this patient's spine and hip?

_____

_____

_____

_____

After immobilizing the patient's spine and injured hip, your partner obtains the patient's blood glucose reading, which is 50 mg/dL. After initiating an IV line of normal saline and administering 25 grams of glucose, the patient's mental status markedly improves. You apply a cardiac monitor, assess the patient's cardiac rhythm **(Figure 12-1)**, and then obtain baseline vital signs and a SAMPLE history **(Table 12-3)**. The neighbor returns with the patient's medications.

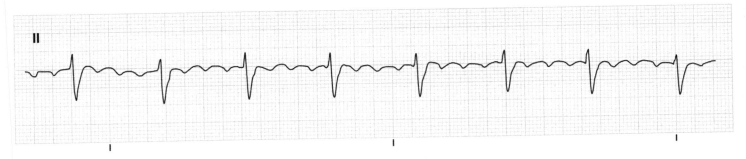

■ **Figure 12-1** Your patient's cardiac rhythm.

Table 12-3 Baseline Vital Signs and SAMPLE History

Blood Pressure	150/90 mm Hg
Pulse	66 beats/min, strong and regular
Respirations	22 breaths/min, adequate tidal volume
Oxygen Saturation	95% (on 100% oxygen)
Signs and Symptoms	Pain to left hip, confusion (resolved)
Allergies	Sulfonamides, Demerol, penicillin
Medications	Vasotec, Calan, Diuril, K-Dur
Pertinent Past History	Atrial flutter, hypertension
Last Oral Intake	"I ate yesterday morning, shortly before I fell."
Events Leading to the Injury	"I slipped on a throw rug while walking into my living room."

The patient is loaded into the ambulance and transport to a local hospital is initiated. Repeat blood glucose analysis reveals a reading of 101 mg/dL. While en route, you talk to the patient and monitor her for signs of deterioration.

4. How does aging affect the body's ability to compensate for shock?

_____

_____

_____

_____

The patient's condition remains stable throughout transport. With an estimated time of arrival at the hospital of 5 minutes, you perform an ongoing assessment **(Table 12-4)** and then call your report to the receiving facility.

Table 12-4 Ongoing Assessment

Level of Consciousness	Conscious and alert to person, place, and time
Airway and Breathing	Airway remains patent; respirations, 20 breaths/min with adequate tidal volume.
Oxygen Saturation	95% (on 100% oxygen)
Blood Pressure	148/86 mm Hg
Pulse	68 beats/min, strong and regular
ECG	Atrial flutter with 4:1 conduction

The patient is delivered to the hospital without incident. Radiographic evaluation confirms a fracture of the left hip. Further examination by the physician reveals no other injuries or illnesses. The patient is admitted to the orthopedic ward, and, after three days, is transferred to a rehabilitation facility.

1. What are common contributing factors to falls in the elderly?

Falls are a common cause of injury in elderly patients and can result in serious problems. According to the American Geriatric Society, fall-related injuries are a leading cause of accidental death in the elderly. Additionally, 50 percent of falls result in lesser injuries (eg, soft tissue trauma), which may not be life-threatening, but can have a profound impact on the patient's quality of life. Children and young adults have a higher incidence of falls than the elderly; however, unlike the elderly, their injuries are not associated with a high mortality rate.

Falls in the elderly are caused by intrinsic (patient related) factors, extrinsic (environmental) factors, or a combination of both (multifactorial). Extrinsic factors include torn or loose rugs, poor lighting, furniture obstructions, wet floors, and high steps on stairways.

Intrinsic factors may be age related or the result of an acute or prior medical condition. Age-related changes include impaired balance and coordination (gait impairment), decreased muscle and bone strength, impaired vision and depth perception, and decreased proprioception (perception of body position and movement).

Common acute medical conditions include myocardial infarction, stroke, hypoglycemia, and infection with associated dehydration. Prior medical illnesses, such as stroke, cataracts, and Parkinson's disease, can impair the elderly patient's balance and coordination, leading to falls.

The use of certain medications can also predispose the elderly patient to falls. These medications include anxiolytics such as temazepam (Restoril) and diazepam (Valium), antidepressants such as amitriptyline (Elavil) and paroxetine (Paxil), and antihypertensives such as propranolol (Inderal) and metoprolol (Lopressor). Medication-related falls are often the result of nervous system impairment, drug-to-drug interaction, or inadvertent overdose. Many elderly patients take multiple medications (polypharmacy) for different medical conditions, and it is often impossible to determine how one drug will interact with another.

The cause of falls in the elderly is often multifactorial. An overmedicated patient may trip on a loose rug or fall down steps or the patient may experience a syncopal episode and strike their head on an end table as they fall. **Table 12-5** summarizes the factors that commonly contribute to falls in the elderly.

Table 12-5 Contributing Factors to Falls in the Elderly

Extrinsic factors
- Torn or loose rugs
- Poor lighting
- Furniture obstructions
- Wet floors
- High steps on stairways

Intrinsic factors
- Age-related changes
  - Impaired balance and coordination
  - Decreased muscle and bone strength
  - Impaired vision or depth perception
  - Impaired proprioception
- Acute medical conditions
  - Myocardial infarction
  - Stroke
  - Hypoglycemia
  - Infection and dehydration
- Prior medical conditions
  - Stroke
  - Cataracts
  - Parkinson's disease
  - Medications (polypharmacy)

Multifactorial
- Fall during a syncopal episode
- Overmedication with resultant fall

Through a careful and systematic assessment of the patient, the paramedic must attempt to determine the cause of the patient's fall. In many cases, a fall may be the only presenting sign of an acute illness. Unfortunately, the patient's fall may be the result of physical abuse, which should be suspected when the injury sustained does not coincide with the mechanism described.

2. What are some common causes of altered mental status in the elderly?

You should assume that any alteration in mental status is abnormal until proven otherwise, regardless of the patient's age. Advanced age does not automatically equate to an altered mental status. Elderly patients are frequently capable of highly creative and productive thought processes.

By the time a person reaches the age of 80, brain size has decreased by approximately 10 percent; however, this decrease in brain size does not affect the person's intelligence. The following slight changes, however, which are not present in all patients, are commonly associated with the aging process:

- Forgetfulness
- Psychomotor slowing
- Decreased reaction time
- Difficulty remembering recent events

When assessing an elderly patient with altered mental status, you must first determine the patient's baseline mental status. According to the neighbor, your patient is normally well oriented. This confirms the presence of a new onset in altered mentation.

Elderly patients are predisposed to several neurological disorders that can produce alterations in mentation. It may not be possible to determine the exact cause in the prehospital setting, which is why these patients should be evaluated in the emergency department. **Table 12-6** lists some of the more common causes of altered mental status in the elderly.

Table 12-6 Common Causes of Altered Mental Status in the Elderly

Cerebrovascular disorders
- Transient ischemic attack
- Stroke

Cardiovascular disorders
- Acute myocardial infarction
- Cardiac dysrhythmias

Postictal phase following a seizure

Medication reactions
- Interactions between multiple drugs
- Underdose or overdose

Infections/Sepsis
- Pneumonia
- Urinary tract infection

Electrolyte disturbances and dehydration

Nutritional deficiencies
- Hypoglycemia
- Deficiency of vitamin B12 (cobalamin)

Thermoregulatory dysfunction
- Hypo- or hyperthermia

Structural abnormalities
- Dementia
- Brain tumor
- Subdural hematoma

Approximately 15 percent of Americans over the age of 65 experience varying degrees of dementia. Dementia is defined as a progressive, irreversible impairment of cognitive function. Alzheimer's disease, a common cause of dementia, is a degenerative disease of the brain that results in impaired memory, thinking, and behavior. Approximately 4.5 million Americans are affected by Alzheimer's disease. Brain tumors, which typically grow slowly, are another possible cause of dementia.

In the prehospital setting, dementia is often difficult to differentiate from delirium, especially in the absence of a friend or family member who is familiar with the patient's normal mental state. Unlike dementia, delirium is characterized by an acute onset of cognitive impairment and is frequently caused by a life-threatening medical condition **(Table 12-7)**. Delirium can be reversed if the underlying cause is rapidly identified and promptly treated.

Table 12-7 Common Causes of Delirium

Acute myocardial infarction or stroke
Drug overdose
Emotional disturbances
Hypoxia
Sepsis
Seizures
Dehydration
Endocrine disorders • Hyper- or hypothyroidism • Hyper- or hypoglycemia
Intracranial hemorrhage • Subdural hematoma

Once it has been established that the altered mental status is a new onset, the paramedic should carefully and systematically assess the patient in an attempt to identify and treat the underlying cause. Routine actions include evaluating for signs of trauma, obtaining a blood glucose reading, and considering the administration of naloxone (Narcan) if a drug overdose is suspected.

Again, do not become complacent and assume that an altered mental status in the elderly patient is simply the result of advanced age.

3. What is kyphosis? How will you immobilize this patient's spine and hip?

Kyphosis is an exaggerated curvature (concave ventral) of the spine that results in a rounded or hunched back **(Figure 12-2)**. Kyphosis can occur for many reasons and at any age; however, in the elderly, it is most commonly caused by osteoporosis. As the bones of the spine weaken and thin, they begin to deteriorate and compress. This results in deformation of the spine, most commonly in the upper thoracic region.

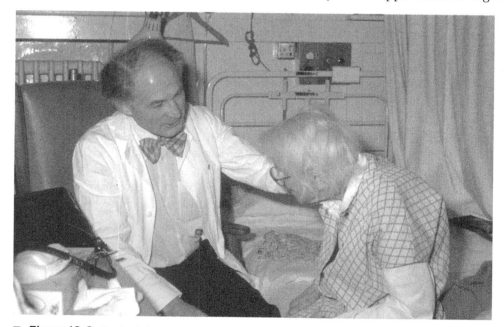

■ **Figure 12-2** Kyphosis is an exaggerated curvature of the spine that results in a rounded or hunched back.

Case Study 12: Answers and Summary

Because of the age-related deterioration of bone structure (eg, osteoporosis), fractures of the spine can occur with even minor mechanisms of injury. Therefore, spinal immobilization of this patient is clearly necessary.

Immobilizing this patient's kyphotic spine will require modification of the spinal immobilization technique. Additionally, as evidenced by the lateral rotation and shortening of her left leg, you should suspect and treat this patient for a hip fracture.

When immobilizing the spine of kyphotic patients, several pillows or blankets may be required to provide support to the head and upper back **(Figure 12-3)**. Padding of these areas is necessary to provide support, because the kyphotic patient's back will not completely conform to the spine board.

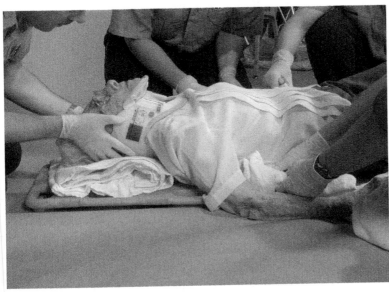

■ **Figure 12-3** Support the head and upper back of the kyphotic patient with pillows and blankets.

Hip fractures are actually fractures of the proximal portion of the femur near or at the site of articulation with the acetabulum **(Figure 12-4)**. Commonly, fractures of the proximal femur can occur in between the femoral head and the trochanteric region (femoral neck fractures), in between the greater and lesser trochanters (intertrochanteric), or below the lesser trochanter (subtrochanteric).

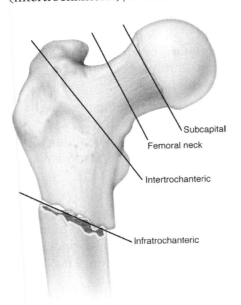

Subcapital
Femoral neck

Intertrochanteric

Infratrochanteric

■ **Figure 12-4** Common hip fracture locations

Hip fractures are commonly splinted by placing pillows or other padding under the injured extremity to support the fracture site in the deformed position **(Figure 12-5)**. Splinting the extremity in the position in which it was found will minimize the risk of further injury as well as reduce the patient's pain.

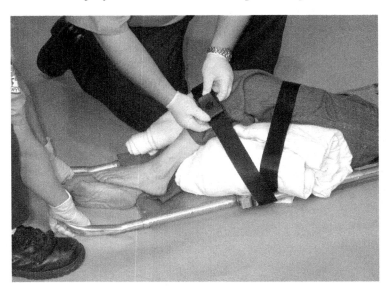

■ **Figure 12-5** Splint a fractured hip in the position found with pillows and blankets.

A long spine board or an orthopedic (scoop) stretcher can be used to immobilize a fractured hip. These devices will allow the patient and the splinting material to be properly secured. Traction splints are not recommended for immobilizing hip fractures. Because it is not possible to determine the exact location of the fracture in the prehospital setting, it is not possible to accurately assess the integrity of the pelvis. If the fracture involves the pelvis, applying a traction splint could actually be detrimental and result in further displacement and potentially injury. Furthermore, the risk of injury to the skin and other soft tissues with the application of traction splints in the elderly is potentially higher. Thus, the use of these devices in elderly hip fracture patients should be avoided unless alternatives are inadequate or otherwise inappropriate.

4. How does aging affect the body's ability to compensate for shock?

Even at rest, the aging body's physiologic functions are diminished. Therefore, the ability of the elderly person to effectively compensate for a low cardiac output, hypoxia, and shock is markedly diminished. The respiratory, nervous, and cardiovascular systems are the key body systems that compensate during shock; therefore, age-related changes that occur with each of these systems will be discussed.

The aging process adversely affects ventilatory function, thus impairing the elderly person's ability to compensate for hypoxia. Smooth muscles of the lower airway weaken with age. When increases in tidal volume are needed (eg, hypoxia, shock), the patient attempts to breath deeply; however, the walls of the lower airway collapse. This reduces tidal volume **(Figure 12-6)**.

Loss of respiratory muscle mass, increases in the stiffness of the thoracic cage, and a decreased surface area available for air exchange contribute to a decrease in vital capacity (volume of air exchanged after maximal inhalation and exhalation) of up to 50 percent. Decreased vital capacity causes an increase in residual volume, which is the amount of air remaining in the lungs following a maximal exhalation. This leaves more stagnant air in the alveoli, which impairs effective gas exchange.

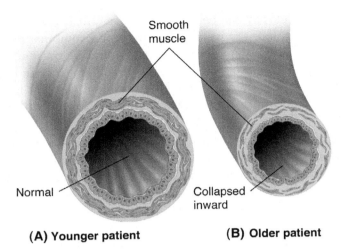

Smooth muscle

Normal

Collapsed inward

(A) Younger patient   **(B) Older patient**

■ **Figure 12-6** (A.) Healthy muscle in the younger patient's airway helps maintain the open airway during the pressures of inhalation. (B.) Muscle weakening with age can lead to airway collapse.

With aging, the body's chemoreceptors become less sensitive. Chemoreceptors, which are located in the aortic arch, sense changes in arterial oxygen and carbon dioxide and send signals to the brainstem to regulate breathing accordingly. Additionally, nerve impulse transmission from the brainstem to the diaphragm and the nerves of the intercostal muscles is decreased. The net effect is a decreased ability to quickly increase respirations in response to conditions that cause hypoxia (ie, shock).

The cardiovascular system undergoes, to varying degrees, age-related deterioration that decreases its ability to compensate for shock. The vasculature loses its elasticity, which causes an increase in systolic blood pressure and afterload (the force that the heart must pump against). As a result, the wall of the left ventricle becomes enlarged (hypertrophy) and thickens. The myocardium also loses its ability to effectively stretch (Frank-Starling effect), thus decreasing ventricular filling and contractility. Hypertrophy of the mitral and tricuspid valves also occurs, which impedes blood flow into and out of the heart. These myocardial changes cause a natural decrease in stroke volume and cardiac output. Furthermore, the ability to increase cardiac output to meet increased demands of the body is decreased.

Baroreceptors, which are located in the aortic arch and carotid sinus, become less sensitive to changes in blood volume with age. These receptors, which sense changes in arterial blood pressure, send messages to the adrenal glands, causing them to secrete the hormones epinephrine and norepinephrine, which causes increases in heart rate, myocardial contractility, and blood pressure. The heart's response to epinephrine and norepinephrine decreases with age; therefore, the elderly person is less able to quickly and effectively compensate for blood loss and decreases in blood volume.

Due to age-related decreases in elastin and collagen in the vascular walls, blood vessel elasticity can be reduced by as much as 70 percent in the elderly person. Therefore, compensation in shock is significantly reduced because the peripheral vasculature must be able to constrict and dilate accordingly to maintain blood pressure and adequate perfusion.

Summary

Falls are a leading cause of accidental death in patients over the age of 65. Contributing factors to falls in the elderly can be intrinsic (eg, age-related changes, acute or prior illness), extrinsic (eg, loose rugs, poor lighting), or a combination of both. When assessing the elderly patient who has fallen, the paramedic must attempt to determine the cause of the fall. Because of osteoporosis, spinal fractures can occur with even minor mechanisms of injury; therefore, the elderly patient who has fallen should be immobilized, with modifications made as needed for the patient with a kyphotic spine.

Hip fractures account for nearly 30 percent of orthopedic hospital admissions each year. Approximately 80 percent of hip fractures occur in women and are most frequently seen in the elderly. The elderly are prone to fractures because of osteoporosis, which makes the bones very fragile. Approximately 20 percent of patients over the age of 65 who are hospitalized for a hip fracture die within the first 6 months following the injury. In the acute setting, death following a hip fracture is usually caused by pneumonia, myocardial infarction, or pulmonary embolus. Long-term, common causes of death include pulmonary embolus and sepsis.

Mental status changes do not occur in all patients with age. Many elderly patients maintain effective cognitive processes. Any change in mentation must be assumed to be abnormal until proven otherwise. The paramedic should determine, by talking with friends or family members, whether the patient's mental status has changed, and, if so, to what degree. Common causes of altered mental status in the elderly include, among others, hypoglycemia, medication-related issues, and stroke. Any patient with an altered mental status should be given supplemental oxygen or assisted ventilations as needed.

Age-related changes reduce the elderly person's ability to quickly and effectively compensate for hemodynamic compromise (eg, blood loss). The muscles of the respiratory system weaken, and the chemoreceptors become less sensitive to changes in oxygen and carbon dioxide levels in the blood. Due to hypertrophy and thickening of the ventricular myocardium, stroke volume decreases, resulting in a decreased cardiac output, both at rest and in times of increased demand. Blood vessel elasticity decreases, making the peripheral vasculature less able to constrict and dilate in response to the body's demands.

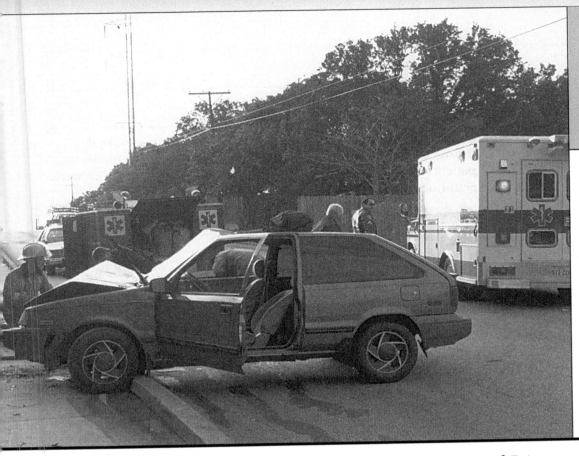

13

32-Year-Old Pregnant Female Involved in a Car Crash

At 9:25 AM, you are dispatched to the corner of Main Street and Brice Lane where a car has struck a utility pole head on. The power company and fire department are also dispatched to the scene. Dispatch advises you that this is a single-patient incident involving a pregnant woman. Your response time to the scene is approximately 5 minutes.

You arrive at the scene at 9:30 AM. The power company has already shut down the power to the utility pole, and a firefighter is maintaining stabilization of the patient's head from the backseat of her car. As you approach the car, you note moderate damage to the front end with airbag deployment. The patient, a 32-year-old female who was driving the vehicle, is still wearing her seatbelt. Your partner retrieves the spinal immobilization equipment while you perform an initial assessment (Table 13-1). The patient is crying and tells you that she is 36 weeks pregnant.

Table 13-1 Initial Assessment

Mechanism of Injury	Single-vehicle crash, auto versus utility pole
Level of Consciousness	Conscious and alert to person, place, and time
Chief Complaint	"My neck and belly hurt. Please save my baby!"
Airway and Breathing	Airway is patent; respirations, increased with adequate tidal volume.
Circulation	Radial pulse is increased, strong, and regular; no gross bleeding noted; skin is pink, warm, and dry.

1. What factors increase maternal and fetal injury severity in a motor-vehicle crash?

_____

_____

_____

After applying a cervical collar and 100% supplemental oxygen, you remove the patient from her car and place her on a long spine board. Because of the moderate damage to the patient's vehicle, her abdominal pain, and the fact that she is 36 weeks pregnant, you perform a rapid trauma assessment **(Table 13-2)**.

Table 13-2 Rapid Trauma Assessment

Head	No obvious trauma
Neck	Trachea is midline; jugular veins, normal; no cervical spine deformities.
Chest	Seatbelt abrasions across the chest; chest wall is stable; breath sounds are clear and equal bilaterally to auscultation.
Abdomen/Pelvis	Abdomen is soft and diffusely tender to palpation; no bruising noted; no vaginal bleeding noted upon visual inspection; pelvis is stable.
Lower Extremities	No obvious trauma; pedal pulses, present bilaterally; sensory and motor functions, grossly intact
Upper Extremities	No obvious trauma; radial pulses, present bilaterally; sensory and motor functions, grossly intact
Posterior	No obvious trauma

Shortly after fully immobilizing the patient's spine, you note a marked decrease in her level of consciousness. Additionally, her skin has become pale and diaphoretic. You immediately reassess the patient to determine the cause of her sudden deterioration.

2. What is the likely cause of this patient's deterioration? What corrective action(s) should you take?

_____

_____

_____

After taking the appropriate corrective action, the patient's condition rapidly improves. You place her onto the stretcher, load her into the ambulance, and obtain baseline vital signs and a SAMPLE history **(Table 13-3)**.

Table 13-3 Baseline Vital Signs and SAMPLE History

Blood Pressure	98/60 mm Hg
Pulse	110 beats/min, strong and regular
Respirations	22 breaths/min, adequate tidal volume
Oxygen Saturation	97% (on 100% oxygen)
Signs and Symptoms	Abdominal tenderness, neck pain
Allergies	None
Medications	Prenatal vitamins
Pertinent Past History	None
Last Oral Intake	Breakfast, approximately 2 hours ago
Events Leading to the Injury	"I lost control of the car when I rounded a corner, and hit the utility pole."

Fetal heart tones are audible with a stethoscope at a rate of 130 beats per minute. You begin transport to a trauma center located 15 miles away. The patient, who remains conscious and alert, tells you that this is her first pregnancy and that she can feel her baby moving.

3. How and why does pregnancy influence the patient's vital sign values?

_____

_____

_____

_____

You place the patient on a cardiac monitor, which displays a sinus tachycardia at 110 beats per minute. After establishing two large-bore IV lines of normal saline, you perform a detailed physical examination **(Table 13-4)**. The patient, still complaining of abdominal pain, remains conscious and alert.

Table 13-4 Detailed Physical Examination

Head and Face	No obvious trauma to the scalp; ears, nose, and mouth are clear; pupils are midpoint, equal, and reactive to light.
Neck	Trachea is midline; jugular veins are normal.
Chest	Seatbelt abrasions across the chest; chest wall is stable; breath sounds are clear and equal bilaterally to auscultation.
Abdomen/Pelvis	Abdomen remains soft but diffusely tender to palpation; no bruising noted; no vaginal bleeding noted upon visual inspection; pelvis is stable.
Lower Extremities	No obvious trauma; pedal pulses, bilaterally present; sensory and motor functions, grossly intact
Upper Extremities	No obvious trauma; radial pulses, bilaterally present; sensory and motor functions, grossly intact
Posterior	Evaluated during the rapid assessment (patient is on a long spine board)

You continuously monitor the patient for signs and symptoms of shock. Your estimated time of arrival at the trauma center is 8 minutes. You provide emotional support to the patient, who is still obviously upset.

4. How would you assess the fetus and uterine fundus in the last trimester of pregnancy?

_____

_____

_____

_____

The patient has remained hemodynamically stable throughout transport. With an estimated time of arrival the hospital of 5 minutes, you perform an ongoing assessment **(Table 13-5)** and then call your radio report to the receiving facility.

Table 13-5 Ongoing Assessment

Level of Consciousness	Conscious and alert to person, place, and time
Airway and Breathing	Airway remains patent; respirations, 22 breaths/min with adequate tidal volume
Oxygen Saturation	98% (on 100% oxygen)
Blood Pressure	90/50 mm Hg
Pulse	90 beats/min, strong and regular
ECG	Normal sinus rhythm

The patient is delivered to the hospital in stable condition. Fetal monitoring is initiated and reveals a fetal heart rate of 140 beats per minute. Assessment of the mother reveals no intraabdominal bleeding or other life-threatening injuries, and radiographic evaluation reveals no injury to her spine. The patient is admitted to labor and delivery for observation and is discharged home the following day.

1. What factors increase maternal and fetal injury severity in a motor-vehicle crash?

As with any patient involved in a motor-vehicle crash, the severity of injury depends on several factors, including the type of impact (eg, front, side, rear, rollover), the speed of the vehicle at the time of impact, and whether the patient was restrained. Because of the anatomic changes that occur during pregnancy, however, the following additional factors increase the risk of significant maternal and fetal injury as a result of a motor-vehicle crash:

- **Direct impact to the abdomen**
  - Because of its anterior protrusion, the pregnant patient's abdomen does not have to travel as far forward before impacting the steering wheel.
  - Direct impact to the gravid (pregnant) uterus clearly increases the risk of maternal intraabdominal hemorrhage and shock, especially beyond the twelfth week of pregnancy.
    - The uterus is protected by the pelvic girdle until the twelfth week of pregnancy, at which time it becomes an abdominal organ and highly susceptible to blunt trauma.
  - Fetal death following blunt abdominal trauma is most often the result of uterine rupture or abruptio placenta, which is a premature separation of the placenta from the uterine wall **(Figure 13-1)**.

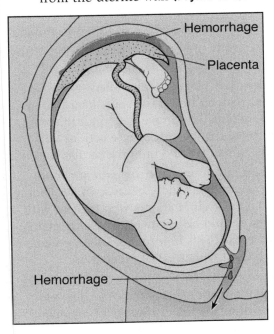

■ **Figure 13-1** With abruptio placenta, the placenta prematurely separates from the uterine wall. Traumatic placental abruption is associated with a high fetal mortality rate.

- **Restraint system use and proper positioning**
  - Seat belt use during pregnancy clearly protects both the mother and the fetus from injury; however, many pregnant women, and others for that matter, do not wear their seat belts properly.
  - Throughout pregnancy, safety belts should be used with *both* the lap belt and shoulder harness in place. The lap belt portion should be placed under the patient's abdomen, over the iliac crests and the symphysis pubis. The shoulder harness should be positioned between the breasts.
  - Placement of the lap belt directly over the abdomen during a deceleration motor-vehicle crash can potentially cause significant uterine, placental, and fetal injury.

Airbags are a secondary or supplemental restraint system (SRS), meaning that they are designed to be used in conjunction with a properly positioned seatbelt. When deployed, airbags displace the force of deceleration between the steering wheel (or dashboard) and the restrained driver, providing added protection. In pregnant patients, airbags are most protective if the seatbelt is properly positioned as previously described and the patient's seat is moved as far back from the steering wheel or dashboard as possible. If the seat is moved too far forward, the force of the deploying airbag can cause trauma to the head, neck, chest, and abdomen, even if the patient is properly restrained with a seatbelt.

When assessing the pregnant patient who has been involved in a motor-vehicle crash, the paramedic should routinely assess the interior of the vehicle, noting specifically the position of the patient's seat, deformities to the steering wheel, anatomic positioning of seatbelts (if used), and whether the airbag deployed.

2. What is the likely cause of this patient's deterioration? What corrective action(s) should you take?

Your patient's deterioration has two possible causes. The most likely cause is a condition known as *supine hypotensive syndrome*. This condition, which most commonly occurs during the third trimester, can occur as early as the twentieth week of pregnancy. Supine hypotensive syndrome is caused by compression of the inferior vena cava by the gravid uterus when the mother is placed in a supine position. Compression of the inferior vena cava results in decreased venous return to the right atrium (preload) and a subsequent drop in cardiac output, which can be substantial.

Patients with supine hypotensive syndrome typically present with hypotension, tachycardia, and other clinical signs of shock (eg, diaphoresis, altered mental status).

Treatment for supine hypotensive syndrome involves placing the mother in the left lateral recumbent position, or, in the case of your patient, tilting the spine board 20 to 30 degrees to the left. If repositioning of the patient fails to improve her condition, you may attempt manual displacement of the uterus to the left side. These actions will relieve the pressure of the gravid uterus off the vena cava and improve cardiac output.

If actions to relieve pressure from the vena cava fail to improve the patient's condition, you should assume that she is bleeding internally; which, because of her abdominal pain, would most likely be intraabdominal in origin. Patients who present with signs of shock and no external signs of trauma should be assumed to be experiencing intraabdominal hemorrhage until proven otherwise. This holds truer in the pregnant patient, especially beyond the twentieth week (first trimester) of pregnancy.

During the first 20 weeks of pregnancy, the uterus is relatively protected from injury by the pelvis, and displacement of the intraabdominal organs is minimal. Therefore, common origins of intraabdominal bleeding within the first 20 weeks of pregnancy include the spleen and liver. Bleeding within the true (anterior) abdominal compartment will produce signs of shock as well as abdominal tenderness, rigidity, distention, and guarding.

Beyond the twentieth week of pregnancy, however, the gravid uterus extends out of the pelvic cavity, displacing the intraabdominal organs toward the diaphragm. At this point, the uterus and urinary bladder become abdominal organs rather than pelvic organs and are more susceptible to injury **(Figure 13-2)**.

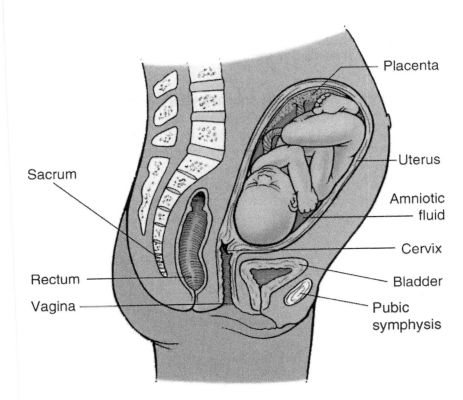

Placenta

Sacrum

Uterus

Amniotic
fluid

Cervix

Rectum

Bladder

Vagina

Pubic
symphysis

■ **Figure 13-2** Beyond the twentieth week of pregnancy, the uterus and urinary bladder become abdominal organs and are more susceptible to injury.

As the uterus progressively enlarges, it becomes protective of the organs in the true abdomen (eg, liver, spleen), providing an "airbaglike" effect; therefore, intraabdominal bleeding beyond the twentieth week of pregnancy commonly occurs in the retroperitoneal space.

The retroperitoneal space, located behind the true abdomen, can accommodate up to 4 liters of blood; therefore, bleeding within this space can be sufficient to produce all of the classic signs of shock (eg, hypotension, tachycardia, diaphoresis, altered mental status). Because the hemorrhage is retroperitoneal, however, the patient may not present with the typical signs of peritoneal irritation (eg, rigidity, guarding, and tenderness) that are commonly seen with hemorrhage in the true abdomen.

Cardiovascular changes during pregnancy can make it difficult for the paramedic to detect internal bleeding. Maternal blood volume increases by as much as 50 percent during pregnancy, which means that the patient can lose as much as 30 to 35 percent of her total blood volume before clinical signs of shock appear. The paramedic, when assessing the injured pregnant patient, must maintain a high index of suspicion for internal hemorrhage, even in the absence of the clinical signs of shock.

Traumatic hemorrhagic shock is clearly life threatening to the mother; however, it is more life threatening to the fetus (mortality rate of approximately 80 percent). The low-resistance blood vessels supplying the uterus constrict vigorously in response to the release of catecholamines (eg, epinephrine, norepinephrine). Therefore, in times of stress, such as during shock, uterine blood flow is reduced. Unfortunately, the uterus cannot increase its own blood supply through vasodilation; therefore, in the early stages of maternal compensatory shock, blood will be diverted away from the uterus (and the fetus). Because maternal hypotension clearly poses grave danger to the fetus, it should be treated aggressively with IV crystalloid fluid boluses and the mother rapidly transported to a trauma center.

If maternal cardiac arrest occurs, begin CPR and follow standard ACLS protocols, including defibrillation for V-Fib and pulseless V-Tach, epinephrine every 3 to 5 minutes, and antidysrhythmic medications if indicated.

3. How and why does pregnancy influence the patient's vital sign values?

A number of physiologic changes occur during pregnancy that influence the patient's vital sign values. During pregnancy, the uterus increases from 2.5 inches to nearly 15 inches in size. Uterine blood flow, which is normally approximately 2 percent of the cardiac output, increases to nearly 20 percent. To accommodate the growing uterus (and fetus), maternal blood volume increases by approximately 50 percent. This causes an increase in the maternal heart rate by 10 to 15 beats/min and a significant increase in cardiac output. The pregnant patient's systolic and diastolic blood pressures typically decrease by 10 to 15 mm Hg.

Blood pressure is an unreliable indicator of perfusion in any patient; however, it is even less reliable in the pregnant patient, because a greater volume of blood can be lost before hypotension develops. Conversely, the paramedic must not assume that lower blood pressures in the pregnant patient are simply a part of the normal physiologic response to pregnancy, especially if the mechanism of injury suggests the potential for internal hemorrhage.

During pregnancy, maternal functional lung capacity and residual volume increase by approximately 20 percent. The cause of this is twofold: elevation of the diaphragm by the enlarging uterus and a 15 percent increase in oxygen use by the placenta, fetus, and maternal organs. To compensate for this decrease in oxygen reserve, increases in maternal respiratory rate, tidal volume, and minute volume occur, which lowers the mother's $PaCO_2$ level. During the third trimester of pregnancy, the mother's $PaCO_2$ is approximately 30 mm Hg (normally 35 to 45 mm Hg in the nonpregnant patient); therefore, she experiences a relative metabolic alkalosis. In response, the kidneys excrete more bicarbonate ions, thus maintaining homeostasis.

During pregnancy, decreased gastric muscle tone reduces gastric motility, with a resultant delay in gastric emptying. Your patient, whose last oral intake was 2 hours prior and who is immobilized to a long spine board, should therefore be presumed to have a full or partially full stomach, which places her at high risk for vomiting and aspiration. You must be prepared to immediately turn the spine board on its side if she begins to vomit.

It must be reemphasized that, although the patient's vital sign values typically change during pregnancy (eg, decreased blood pressure, increased heart rate, increased respirations), the paramedic must not assume this to be "normal" and discount the possibility of shock. Treatment for the mother should be based on her symptomatology and the mechanism of injury. Hemodynamic compromise in the mother will undoubtedly result in decreased perfusion to the fetus.

4. How would you assess the fetus and uterine fundus in the last trimester of pregnancy?

Clearly, the abdominal examination in a pregnant patient will differ from that of the nontrauma patient. After stabilizing life-threatening problems (eg, airway compromise, severe bleeding) in the mother, the paramedic should then perform an obstetric examination, which includes palpation of the uterine fundus (top of the uterus), a quick visual inspection for vaginal bleeding or discharge, and evaluation of fetal heart tones. The goal of the obstetric assessment is to determine the presence of uteroplacental injury and/or fetal distress.

By the third trimester of pregnancy, the uterine fundus should present as a well-defined dome that is easily palpated. An asymmetrical or poorly defined uterine fundus may indicate uterine rupture and intraabdominal bleeding. Additionally, a rigid or tender uterus could indicate uteroplacental injury, such as abruptio placenta.

Fetal age in weeks can be estimated by measuring the distance in centimeters between the symphysis pubis bone and the dome of the uterine fundus. In your patient, who is 36 weeks pregnant, the fundus should be approximately 1 inch below the xiphoid process.

When palpating the uterine fundus, note its shape (ie, symmetrical, asymmetrical) and the presence of fetal movement. During the third trimester, the fetus should be engaged; meaning that it should be in a head-down (cephalic) position, in preparation for delivery. Therefore, kicking movements of the fetus should be palpated at or near the fundus. Additionally, you should ask the mother when she last felt the baby move. The absence of fetal movement following abdominal trauma is an ominous sign.

Auscultating fetal heart tones in the field can be difficult; however, during the last month of pregnancy, they can usually be auscultated with an ordinary stethoscope. Some EMS systems carry Doppler devices for this purpose. To auscultate fetal heart tones, place the bell of the stethoscope firmly in the periumbilical area, which is the area surrounding the umbilicus. The normal fetal heart rate ranges from 120 to 160 beats per minute. In early fetal distress, the heart rate may exceed 160 beats per minute. Sustained bradycardia (less than 100 beats/min), however, is an ominous sign that may indicate abruptio placenta, hypoxia, or fetal brain injury.

As previously discussed, early maternal compensation for shock causes the diversion of blood away from the uterus. When this occurs, fetal blood supply is compromised and the fetus becomes distressed (tachycardia or bradycardia). Therefore, fetal distress often presents before the typical early signs of maternal shock appear (eg, diaphoresis, altered mental status). Fetal heart rate should be considered another vital sign in evaluating the hemodynamic status of the mother.

Summary

When assessing and managing the pregnant patient, the paramedic must remember that he or she is assessing and managing two patients, especially if the patient is beyond 28 weeks gestation, at which point the fetus is considered to be viable and capable of surviving outside of the uterus.

Trauma during pregnancy is most commonly the result of blunt abdominal injury following a motor-vehicle crash; however, the pregnant patient also is subject to the same types of injuries as the nonpregnant patient, including gunshot wounds and falls.

Abruptio placenta and uterine rupture, which pose a greater threat to the fetus than to the mother, are complications associated with blunt abdominal trauma. Beyond the twentieth week of pregnancy, intraabdominal bleeding is usually retroperitoneal and may not present with the signs commonly associated with bleeding into the true abdomen (eg, bruising, rigidity, distention, tenderness).

In assessing and managing the pregnant patient, the paramedic must consider the physiologic changes that occur during pregnancy and how they affect vital sign values. However, maintenance of a high index of suspicion and careful evaluation of the mechanism of injury are often more sensitive predictors of maternal and fetal injury than the patient's vital signs.

Fetal mortality is directly related to maternal mortality; therefore, maximizing the chances of maternal survival will maximize fetal survival. Management for the pregnant trauma patient includes administering 100% supplemental oxygen or assisted ventilations if needed, spinal immobilization with the board tilted to the left to prevent supine hypotensive syndrome, IV crystalloid infusions to maintain maternal blood pressure, and rapid transport to a trauma center.

Should cardiac arrest occur in the mother, follow standard ACLS protocols, including defibrillation for V-Fib or pulseless V-Tach, epinephrine every 3 to 5 minutes, and antidysrhythmic medications if indicated.

14

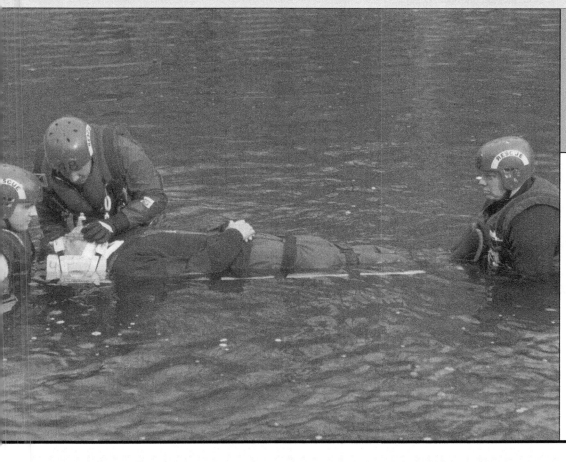

18-Year-Old Male Near-Drowning Victim

At 5:15 PM, you are dispatched to a river at the city park for a possible drowning. Your department's water rescue team is simultaneously dispatched. The temperature outside is 45°F, and your response time to the scene is 6 minutes.

Upon your arrival, rescue personnel are providing mouth-to-mask ventilations on the patient, an 18-year-old male. The patient was apparently submerged for approximately 10 minutes before being rescued. Rescue personnel have removed the patient's wet clothing, placed blankets on him, and have fully immobilized his spine. After quickly and carefully moving the patient into the warm ambulance, you perform an initial assessment **(Table 14-1)**.

Table 14-1 Initial Assessment

Mechanism of Injury	Submersion injury
Level of Consciousness	Unconscious and unresponsive
Chief Complaint	Unconscious and apneic
Airway and Breathing	Airway is patent; respirations, absent.
Circulation	Pulse is slow, weak, and regular; skin, cold and wet; no gross bleeding noted.

1. What is the pathophysiology of drowning and near-drowning?

_____

_____

_____

Your partner suctions secretions from the patient's oropharynx, inserts an oropharyngeal airway, and, with a rescue member's assistance, continues ventilations with a BVM device and 100% oxygen. No one witnessed the patient's submersion; however, according to a bystander, the patient had been seen consuming alcohol prior to the event.

2. How can hypothermia affect the outcome of a near-drowning patient?

_____

_____

_____

After your partner successfully intubates the patient, a rescue member continues ventilations with 100% oxygen. A nasogastric tube is inserted to evacuate water from the patient's stomach. After obtaining the patient's core body temperature, which is 89°F, you perform a rapid trauma assessment **(Table 14-2)**. Your partner attaches the cardiac monitor, which reveals a sinus bradycardia at 40 beats per minute **(Figure 14-1)**.

Table 14-2 Rapid Trauma Assessment

Head	Contusion to the forehead, no other trauma noted
Neck	Trachea, midline; jugular veins, normal; no cervical spine deformities
Chest	No obvious trauma; chest is stable and symmetrical; breath sounds, clear and equal bilaterally to auscultation.
Abdomen/Pelvis	Abdomen, soft and nontender; pelvis, stable
Lower Extremities	No obvious trauma; pedal pulses, absent; unable to assess sensory and motor functions
Upper Extremities	No obvious trauma; radial pulses, absent; unable to assess sensory and motor functions
Posterior	Unable to assess (patient is immobilized); rescue members state that no injury was present during their assessment.

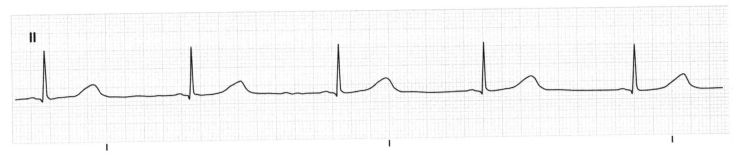

■ **Figure 14-1** Your patient's cardiac rhythm displays a sinus bradycardia at 40 beats per minute.

3. What specific treatment is required for this patient?

_____

_____

_____

_____

4. What is rewarming shock?

_____

_____

_____

_____

You establish an IV and, per medical control, infuse warmed normal saline at a rate of 125 mL/hr. Because your partner's assistance is needed for appropriate patient care, you ask a rescue member to drive the ambulance. Shortly before departing the scene, you obtain a set of baseline vital signs **(Table 14-3)**. Because the patient is unconscious and no family members or friends are present, you are unable to obtain information for the SAMPLE history.

Table 14-3 Baseline Vital Signs and SAMPLE History

Blood Pressure	80/40 mm Hg (difficult to auscultate)
Pulse	44 beats/min, weak and regular
Respirations	Absent (intubated and ventilated with 100% warmed oxygen)
Oxygen Saturation	Unable to assess due to poor extremity perfusion
Signs and Symptoms	Unconscious, apnea, hypotension, bradycardia, contusion to the forehead
Allergies	Unknown
Medications	Unknown
Pertinent Past History	Unknown
Last Oral Intake	Unknown
Events Leading to the Injury	Fell into cold water after drinking alcohol

Transport to a hospital 20 miles away is initiated. En route, efforts are continued to carefully raise the patient's core body temperature. Your partner continues ventilatory support while you perform a detailed physical examination **(Table 14-4)**.

Table 14-4 Detailed Physical Examination

Head and Face	Contusion to the forehead; ears, nose, and mouth are clear; pupils are dilated and sluggishly reactive to light.
Neck	Trachea, midline; jugular veins, normal
Chest	No obvious trauma; chest wall, stable and symmetrical; breath sounds, clear and equal bilaterally to auscultation
Abdomen/Pelvis	Abdomen, soft; pelvis, stable
Lower Extremities	No obvious trauma; pedal pulses, absent
Upper Extremities	No obvious trauma; radial pulses, weakly present
Posterior	Unable to examine (patient is on a long spine board)

You reassess the patient's core body temperature and note that it has increased to 91°F. The cardiac monitor is displaying a sinus rhythm at 65 beats per minute. Your partner advises you that the patient is attempting occasional respiratory effort. After performing an ongoing assessment **(Table 14-5)**, you call your radio report to the receiving facility.

Table 14-5 Ongoing Assessment

Level of Consciousness	Responsive to painful stimuli
Airway and Breathing	Intubated; spontaneous respiratory effort noted
Oxygen Saturation	97% (intubated and ventilated with 100% oxygen)
Blood Pressure	90/60 mm Hg
Pulse	64 beats/min, stronger and regular
ECG	Normal sinus rhythm

5. What secondary complications can occur following a near-drowning?

_____

_____

_____

_____

You arrive at the receiving hospital and transfer care of the patient to the attending physician. Additional rewarming interventions are performed in the emergency department. The patient's level of consciousness improves, and he is now beginning to resist the endotracheal tube. Following sedation with the appropriate medication, a chest radiograph is obtained, which reveals a small amount of water in the patient's lungs. The patient is admitted to the medical intensive care unit, where he later recovered.

1. What is the pathophysiology of drowning and near-drowning?

In drownings and near-drownings (also referred to as submersion injuries), asphyxiation occurs due to submersion in a liquid medium, usually water. A drowning occurs when a submersion victim fails to regain or maintain spontaneous respirations and a pulse following initial resuscitative efforts. A near-drowning occurs when a patient regains and maintains spontaneous respirations and a pulse for greater than 24 hours following resuscitation. It should be noted, however, that not all near-drowning victims survive. Death beyond 24 hours may occur due to secondary complications, which will be discussed later in this case study.

Drownings are a leading cause of death in all age groups. According to the Centers for Disease Control and Prevention (CDC), drowning is the second leading cause of injury-related death in children between 1 and 14 years of age; 80 percent of these young victims are males. Alcohol use is associated with approximately 25 to 50 percent of drownings involving the adolescent and adult age groups.

Drownings typically occur when a person who cannot swim falls into the water or when something goes wrong when a person is already in the water (eg, entanglement, trauma). Initially, the patient panics and begins swallowing large amounts of water. At the same time, the patient makes panicked attempts to inhale, which leads to inadequate breathing, hypoxia, and hypercarbia.

Eventually, the patient experiences decreased buoyancy, becomes exhausted, and then falls below the water's surface. If not removed quickly from the water, respiratory and cardiac arrest will rapidly occur. **Figure 14-2** summarizes the sequence of events that typically precede a drowning.

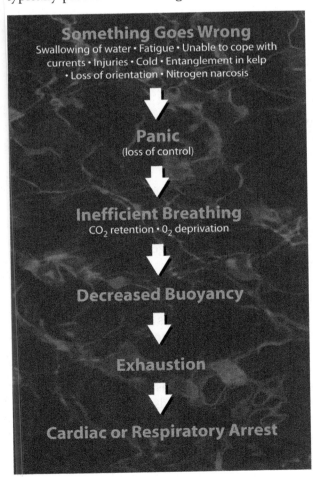

Something Goes Wrong
Swallowing of water • Fatigue • Unable to cope with currents • Injuries • Cold • Entanglement in kelp • Loss of orientation • Nitrogen narcosis

Panic
(loss of control)

Inefficient Breathing
CO_2 retention • O_2 deprivation

Decreased Buoyancy

Exhaustion

Cardiac or Respiratory Arrest

■ **Figure 14-2**
The sequence of events preceding a drowning

In approximately 15 percent of drowning victims, and in a greater percentage of near-drowning victims, laryngospasm occurs due to aspiration of even a small amount of water. Laryngospasm prevents water from entering the lungs, resulting in what is referred to as a "dry" drowning. If laryngospasm does not occur, water freely enters the lungs, resulting in a "wet" drowning. In 85 to 90 percent of cases, significant amounts of water enter the lungs of the drowning victim.

If water enters the lungs (wet drowning), physiologic reactions vary based on the tonicity of the water that the patient was submerged in. In other words, different intrapulmonary complications occur in fresh-water than in salt-water drownings.

Fresh water is hypotonic to blood plasma. Because of the large surface area of the alveoli and bronchioles, fresh water diffuses across the alveolar/capillary membrane and into the vascular space. This causes an increase in blood plasma volume with a relative decrease in red blood cell concentration (hemodilution). Fresh-water drowning also causes alveolar wall thickening, bleeding within the parenchyma of the lungs (hemorrhagic pneumonitis), and the destruction of pulmonary surfactant.

Pulmonary surfactant is a lubricant that lines the alveolar walls and decreases surface tension (keeping the alveoli open). In the absence of pulmonary surfactant, alveolar collapse (atelectasis) and pulmonary shunting occur. During pulmonary shunting, damaged alveoli prevent reoxygenation of the blood (blood bypasses the alveoli); therefore, it is returned, unoxygenated, back to the systemic circulation.

Salt water, which is nearly five times more hypertonic than blood plasma, draws water from the circulatory system into the alveoli, causing pulmonary edema and profound pulmonary shunting. This results in failure of oxygenation and severe hypoxemia. Additionally, because of CO_2 retention and anaerobic metabolism (lactic acid production), respiratory and metabolic acidosis develops.

It is important to note that regardless of the circumstance in which the drowning or near-drowning occurs (ie, wet versus dry drowning, fresh versus salt water), the end result is the same—impaired oxygenation and ventilation and hypoxemia. Prehospital management, therefore, is the same regardless of the circumstance and focuses on aggressive oxygenation and ventilation.

2. How can hypothermia affect the outcome of a near-drowning patient?

Typically, brain death occurs after approximately 4 to 6 minutes without oxygen; however, this rule does not necessarily apply to patients who are submerged in cold water (less than 70°F).

If hypothermia occurs *before* hypoxia, the heart and brain can remain viable well beyond 6 minutes. Therefore, resuscitation from cardiac arrest may be possible, even in cases when the patient has been submerged for up to 30 minutes or longer. However, patients who are submerged for 60 minutes or longer, even in the presence of hypothermia, are rarely resuscitated.

The mammalian diving reflex is an important contributor to survival following submersion in cold water. Following submersion in cold water, breathing is inhibited, bradycardia develops, and, through vasoconstriction, blood is diverted away from tissues that are relatively tolerant of hypoxia (eg, bowel, skin) toward the heart and brain. The colder the water, the more blood flow is diverted to the heart and brain. Additionally, oxygen demand is decreased secondary to a decrease in metabolism. As a result of these processes, oxygen is sent to and used in areas that are most needed to sustain life, thus allowing them to withstand longer periods of hypoxemia. The mammalian diving reflex is most effective in children and young adults; however, because of the physiologic changes associated with aging, it is much less effective in older adults and the elderly.

Cold-water drownings are the source of the adage, "The patient is not dead until he or she is warm and dead." The hypothermic patient may appear to be dead; however, the heart and brain, because of markedly decreased metabolic demands, may be responsive to resuscitation.

3. What specific treatment is required for this patient?

Although your patient has already been removed from the water, it should be emphasized that water rescue should *only* be attempted by trained personnel. Additionally, because the circumstances surrounding your patient's submersion are unclear, spinal injury must be assumed, and the patient's spine should be fully immobilized.

Your patient is apneic; therefore, positive pressure ventilations should be performed. The use of cricoid pressure (Sellick's maneuver) can reduce the risk of further gastric distention and regurgitation with possible aspiration. After preoxygenating the patient for 2 to 3 minutes, the patient's airway should be secured with an endotracheal tube and ventilations continued with warmed humidified oxygen, if available. If local protocols permit, a nasogastric tube should be inserted for gastric decompression.

The following interventions, many of which have already been performed on your patient, should be carried out on *all* hypothermic patients:

- **Remove wet clothing and protect from further heat loss.**
- **Avoid rough handling and excessive activity.**
  - The hypothermic myocardium is extremely irritable and highly susceptible to ventricular fibrillation.
    - Defibrillation and cardiac medications (eg, epinephrine, lidocaine) are typically not effective in treating ventricular fibrillation or pulseless ventricular tachycardia associated with severe hypothermia (≤86°F).
- **Monitor core body temperature.**
  - Hypothermia is defined as being mild, moderate, or severe.
    - Mild: 93.2°F to 96.8° F (34°C to 36°C)
    - Moderate: 86°F to 93.2°F (30°C to 34°C)
    - Severe: Less than 86°F (30°C)
- **Monitor cardiac rhythm.**

Your patient has a core body temperature of 89°F (moderate hypothermia). According to the American Heart Association, moderate hypothermia is treated with passive external rewarming and active external rewarming of the *truncal areas only*. However, because active external rewarming can cause rewarming shock, it is generally not recommended in the prehospital setting unless transport time to the hospital will be delayed and medical control authorizes it.

Passive external rewarming involves placing warm blankets or other insulation barriers on the patient, thus allowing the patient's core body temperature to rise gradually and naturally.

Active external rewarming, if performed, involves placing heat packs to areas of high heat transfer, such as the groin, axillae, and the base of the neck.

4. What is rewarming shock?

Rewarming shock is a potential complication of active external rewarming of the body following hypothermia. Rewarming shock occurs when external heat is applied to the body. As a result, a reflex vasodilation occurs and shunts cold blood and anaerobic metabolism byproducts (eg, lactic acid) to the core of the body.

Rewarming shock causes a paradoxical drop in core body temperature, which leads to worsened core hypothermia, hypotension, and perhaps even cardiac arrest. If active external rewarming is performed, concomitant administration of warmed IV crystalloid fluids (95°F to 100°F) may help to prevent rewarming shock.

You should adhere to locally established protocols and/or contact medical control as needed regarding the prehospital rewarming of the hypothermic patient.

5. What secondary complications can occur following a near-drowning?

Approximately 90 percent of near-drowning patients survive their submersion injury without any residual or secondary effects. Nonetheless, the near-drowning patient, even if fully resuscitated at the scene, should be transported to the hospital, because life-threatening secondary complications can develop 24 hours or more after the incident.

The most common secondary complications following a near-drowning event are aspiration pneumonia, pulmonary edema, pulmonary insufficiency, and adult respiratory distress syndrome (ARDS). Other complications include renal failure, myocardial infarction, and stroke.

ARDS is a life-threatening complication than can occur following a near-drowning and is associated with a very high mortality rate. Any respiratory system insult can result in the development of ARDS; the condition is not exclusive to the near-drowning patient. Because of the physiologic stress associated with near-drowning, the lungs can leak fluid into the alveoli, causing severe inflammation, alveolar destruction, and respiratory system failure. ARDS usually occurs within 24 to 48 hours of the injury or illness.

Signs of secondary pulmonary complications (including ARDS) associated with near-drowning include increasing dyspnea, hemoptysis (coughing up of pink frothy sputum), cyanosis, and alterations in mental status.

Summary

Drownings are a leading cause of death in all age groups. Drowning is the second leading cause of injury-related death in children between 1 and 14 years of age; 80 percent of these young victims are males. Alcohol use is associated with 25 to 50 percent of all drownings and near-drownings in the adolescent and adult age groups. Spinal injury secondary to falls or diving injuries are commonly associated with water-related incidents.

Drowning occurs when a submersion victim fails to regain or maintain spontaneous respirations and a pulse following initial resuscitative efforts. A near-drowning occurs when the submersion victim regains and maintains spontaneous respirations and a pulse for greater than 24 hours following resuscitation. However, death beyond 24 hours may occur as the result of pulmonary or other complications.

Hypothermia is often associated with drownings and near-drownings, especially when the water is 70°F or colder. Hypothermia can protect the heart and brain, especially if it occurs before hypoxia. The mammalian diving reflex, decreased metabolism, and decreased oxygen demand may allow vital organs to survive longer periods of hypoxemia before sustaining permanent damage. Children and young adults have been fully resuscitated following submersion of up to 30 minutes in cold water.

After the patient has been removed from the water by trained personnel, treatment for the drowning or near-drowning patient involves spinal immobilization, aggressive airway management, thermal management, and prompt transport. Water rescue should not be attempted by nontrained personnel.

The oropharynx should be suctioned as needed, and, if local protocol permits, a nasogastric tube should be inserted to evacuate water from the stomach. Provide ventilatory support as needed and secure the unconscious patient's airway with an endotracheal tube.

Hypothermia should be treated with passive external rewarming and the infusion of warmed IV crystalloid fluids. Active external rewarming, because of the risk of rewarming shock, is generally not recommended in the field; however, if transport times are lengthy and medical control authorizes it, chemical heat packs may be placed in the axillae, at the base of the neck, and over the groin.

The hypothermic patient must be handled very carefully, because the cold myocardium is highly susceptible to ventricular fibrillation. Cardiac arrest associated with a core body temperature of 86°F or lower is typically unresponsive to defibrillation and cardiac medications.

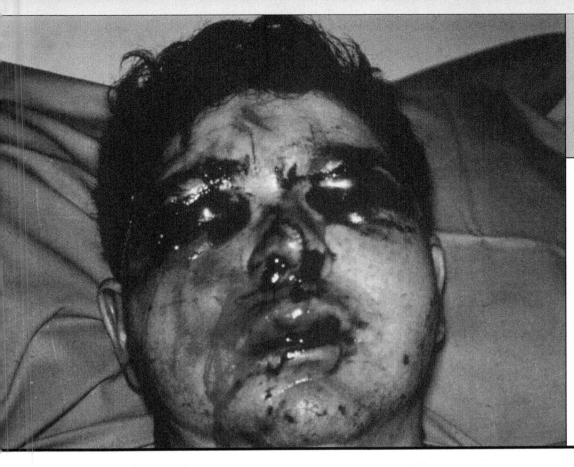

15

25-Year-Old Male with Severe Maxillofacial Trauma

At 1:40 AM, law enforcement requests your assistance for a 25-year-old male who was attacked and severely beaten by a rival gang. You proceed to the scene, which is approximately 7 minutes from your station. En route, an on-scene police officer advises you that the scene is secure and that the patient is unconscious.

You arrive at the scene at 1:47 AM. You find the patient lying unconscious in a supine position. As you approach him, you note that he has massive maxillofacial trauma and gurgling respirations. Your partner assumes manual in-line stabilization of the patient's head while you perform an initial assessment **(Table 15-1)**. You ask a police officer to call for additional EMS assistance.

Table 15-1 Initial Assessment

Mechanism of Injury	Blunt facial trauma
Level of Consciousness	Unconscious and unresponsive
Chief Complaint	Unconscious, massive facial trauma
Airway and Breathing	Respirations are rapid, shallow, and gurgling; blood is noted in the oropharynx.
Circulation	Pulse, rapid and weak; skin, cool and clammy; blood coming from the mouth, ears, and nose; no other gross bleeding

1. What immediate care must you provide for this patient?

_____

_____

_____

_____

Your partner stabilizes the patient's head with his knees and initiates appropriate airway management. Another paramedic crew was in the immediate area and arrives shortly after your call for assistance. You perform a rapid trauma assessment (Table 15-2) while an assisting paramedic helps your partner manage the patient's airway.

Table 15-2 Rapid Trauma Assessment

Head	Severe swelling and multiple contusions to the face; bleeding from the mouth, nose, and ears
Neck	Trachea is midline; jugular veins, normal; no cervical spine deformities.
Chest	No obvious trauma; chest wall, stable and symmetrical; breath sounds are diminished bilaterally, but equal.
Abdomen/Pelvis	Abdomen, soft and nontender; pelvis, stable
Lower Extremities	No obvious trauma; pedal pulses, weakly present; unable to assess sensory and motor functions
Upper Extremities	No obvious trauma; radial pulses, weakly present; unable to assess sensory and motor functions
Posterior	No obvious trauma

Your partner is having difficulty ventilating the patient with the BVM. Preparations for endotracheal intubation are made while an assisting paramedic retrieves the spinal immobilization equipment and stretcher from the ambulance. A cardiac monitor is attached to the patient and reveals a sinus tachycardia at 110 beats per minute. The patient's oxygen saturation is 89% while being ventilated with a BVM.

2. What problems should be anticipated when intubating this patient?

_____

_____

_____

_____

After preoxygenating the patient, your partner attempts endotracheal intubation while an assisting paramedic maintains manual in-line stabilization of the patient's head. However, because of the patient's massive facial trauma, unstable mandible, and oropharyngeal bleeding, the paramedic is unable to view the vocal cords. BVM ventilations and suctioning are continued.

3. Is a dual-lumen airway device a viable alternative for this patient? Why or why not?

_____

_____

_____

_____

The patient's spine is fully immobilized, and he is quickly loaded into the ambulance. Your partner and the paramedic assistant continue aggressive airway management. The patient's brother, who was notified by law enforcement, arrives at the scene and is able to provide you with the patient's medical information. You quickly obtain baseline vital signs and a SAMPLE history **(Table 15-3)**, at which time transport to a trauma center is begun.

En route to the trauma center, two more attempts at intubation fail. You and your partner agree that a cricothyrotomy, which is authorized by your protocols, must be performed. Your partner continues oropharyngeal suctioning and BVM ventilations while you prepare the necessary equipment.

Table 15-3 Baseline Vital Signs and SAMPLE History

Blood Pressure	160/90 mm Hg
Pulse	110 beats/min, weak and regular
Respirations	30 breaths/min, shallow and gurgling (Oropharyngeal suctioning and BVM ventilations are being performed.)
Oxygen Saturation	89% (with ventilations and 100% oxygen)
Signs and Symptoms	Unconscious, severe maxillofacial trauma, unstable mandible, oropharyngeal bleeding, inadequate breathing
Allergies	None
Medications	None
Pertinent Past History	None
Last Oral Intake	According to the brother, "We ate supper together about 3 hours ago."
Events Leading to the Injury	A rival gang apparently attacked the patient.

4. What are the two types of cricothyrotomy? When are they indicated?

_____

_____

_____

_____

After successfully performing a cricothyrotomy, the patient's airway is secured and ventilations with a BVM device are continued. Oropharyngeal suctioning is continued as needed to keep the patient's airway clear of blood. After establishing an IV line of normal saline, you perform an ongoing assessment **(Table 15-4)**. With an estimated time of arrival at the trauma center of 5 minutes, you call your radio report to the receiving facility.

Table 15-4 Ongoing Assessment

Level of Consciousness	Unconscious and unresponsive
Airway and Breathing	Airway secured by cricothyrotomy, ventilated at a rate of 15 breaths/min with a BVM device and 100% oxygen
Oxygen Saturation	96% (ventilated with 100% oxygen)
Blood Pressure	150/86 mm Hg
Pulse	100 beats/min, stronger and regular
ECG	Sinus tachycardia

The patient is delivered to the trauma center, where aggressive treatment is continued. A computer tomographic (CT) scan of the patient's head reveals a fracture of the basilar skull and massive intracranial bleeding. After being stabilized in the emergency department, he is taken to surgery. Unfortunately, however, the patient died the next day.

CASE STUDY ANSWERS AND SUMMARY

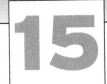

1. What immediate care must you provide for this patient?

Your patient's airway is in jeopardy and requires immediate, aggressive management. A patent airway must first be established by suctioning the blood from the patient's oropharynx. Until a patent airway is established, further management (i.e., attempting ventilation) would be futile. Once the airway has been cleared of blood, an airway adjunct must be inserted. Because the patient is unconscious and unresponsive, an oropharyngeal airway should be inserted. The blood draining from the patient's nose should be assumed to contain cerebrospinal fluid (cerebrospinal rhinnorhea) and is suggestive of a fracture of the cribriform plate; therefore, nasopharyngeal airway insertion is contraindicated.

Because his respirations are rapid and shallow, tidal volume and minute volume are both reduced. Therefore, ventilatory assistance with a BVM (or pocket mask) device and 100% oxygen will be required.

Airway management can be problematic in patients with massive maxillofacial trauma, because there are often multiple problems that require simultaneous care. Your patient is a perfect example of this type of situation, because his airway is obstructed by blood in the oropharynx and his breathing is inadequate. This situation is most effectively managed by providing oropharyngeal suctioning for 15 seconds and then ventilating the patient for 2 minutes.

This alternating pattern of suctioning and ventilating should continue until the airway is clear of blood or the airway has been definitively secured. It is clear that this patient is going to require advanced airway management; therefore, preparations for endotracheal intubation should be made.

2. What problems should be anticipated when intubating this patient?

Airway management in patients with severe maxillofacial trauma can be challenging. With this patient, several complicating factors should be anticipated that will make it difficult to perform the intubation.

First and foremost, the continuous oropharyngeal bleeding is going to obscure your view of the anatomic landmarks that must be viewed during intubation (ie, epiglottis, vocal cords); therefore, frequent suctioning will be required both during and between intubation attempts. Additionally, broken teeth are likely to be encountered; they must be removed before they obstruct the upper airway or are aspirated into the lungs. To avoid worsened hypoxia, preoxygenation with a BVM both before and after suctioning, as well as between intubation attempts, is essential.

Instability of the patient's fractured mandible is going to further complicate endotracheal intubation. When performing laryngoscopy, a stable mandible is necessary to allow you to achieve an adequate view of the epiglottis and vocal cords. Additionally, mandibular fractures can cause tetanic muscle spasms of the jaw (trismus), making it difficult to open the patient's mouth. In such cases, pharmacologic interventions (eg, sedation, neuromuscular blockade) may be required to facilitate intubation.

Because this patient has sustained severe maxillofacial trauma, spinal injury must be assumed as well; therefore, intubation must be performed with the patient's head in a neutral in-line position.

The patient should be attached to a cardiac monitor and a pulse oximeter during the intubation attempt. The intubation attempt should be aborted after 30 seconds, if the oxygen saturation falls below 90%, or the patient experiences significant heart rate or cardiac rhythm changes. If the intubation attempt must be aborted, ventilate the patient with 100% oxygen at a rate of 24 breaths per minute for 2 to 3 minutes.

Repeated intubation attempts will generally not harm the patient; however, individual prolonged attempts will.

3. Is a dual-lumen airway device a viable alternative for this patient? Why or why not?

Dual-lumen airway devices, such as the esophageal Combitube and Pharyngotracheal Lumen Airway (Figure 15-1), would be of minimal benefit for this particular patient.

Because dual-lumen airway devices are inserted blindly into the airway, they come to rest in the esophagus in the vast majority of cases. Although this would facilitate air flow into the lungs, the airway would still be vulnerable to aspiration because of the patient's ongoing oropharyngeal bleeding.

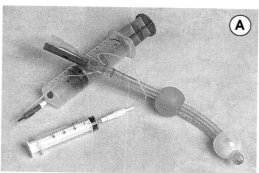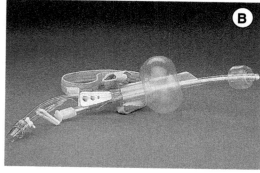

■ **Figure 15-1** (A.) The Combitube and (B.) the Pharyngotracheal Lumen Airway. These devices will not protect the airway from aspiration. Because they are inserted blindly, they usually come to rest in the esophagus, leaving the trachea and lungs unprotected.

4. What are the two types of cricothyrotomy? When are they indicated?

Cricothyrotomy is an emergency airway procedure that is performed when a patent airway cannot be established with conventional methods (eg, BVM ventilation, intubation). Cricothyrotomy provides a rapid means of obtaining a patent airway, using the cricothyroid membrane as a direct entry point into the trachea (Figure 15-2).

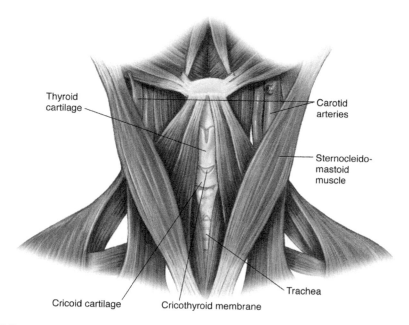

■ **Figure 15-2** The cricothyroid membrane is a direct entry point into the trachea.

Relative to less-invasive airway management techniques, more complications are associated with cricothyrotomy; therefore, it is usually performed as a measure of last resort. If the airway can be secured by other means (basic or advanced), cricothyrotomy is not indicated. There are two type of cricothyrotomies: surgical and needle.

A surgical cricothyrotomy, also referred to as an open cricothyrotomy, involves vertically incising the cricothyroid membrane with a scalpel and inserting an endotracheal tube or tracheostomy tube through the cricothyroid membrane and directly into the trachea **(Figure 15-3)**. A BVM device or automatic ventilator is then attached to the tube to provide effective ventilations.

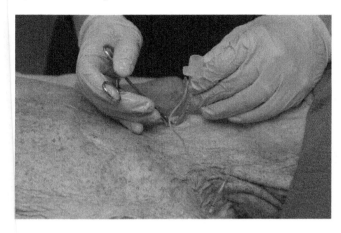

■ **Figure 15-3** A surgical cricothyrotomy involves incising the cricothyroid membrane and inserting an endotracheal tube or tracheostomy tube directly into the trachea.

A needle cricothyrotomy also uses the cricothyroid membrane as an entry point into the trachea; however, instead of incising the cricothyroid membrane, a large-bore (14- to 16-gauge) IV catheter is inserted through the cricothyroid membrane and into the trachea **(Figure 15-4)**. Ventilations are then provided by attaching a high-pressure jet ventilator to the hub of the IV catheter. Although the open cricothyrotomy is preferred over the needle cricothyrotomy, locally established protocol should be followed regarding which procedure (if either) you are authorized to perform.

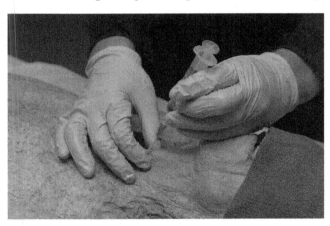

■ **Figure 15-4** A needle cricothyrotomy involves inserting a large-bore IV catheter through the cricothyroid membrane and into the trachea.

As previously discussed, cricothyrotomy is indicated when all attempts to secure a patent airway with less-invasive techniques have failed. This is clearly the case with your patient, whose massive maxillofacial trauma and continued oropharyngeal bleeding have prevented you from effectively ventilating and intubating him. **Table 15-5** summarizes the indications for performing a cricothyrotomy.

Table 15-5 Indications for performing a cricothyrotomy

Severe maxillofacial trauma

- Severe maxillofacial trauma is often accompanied by a fractured maxilla and/or mandible, which makes BVM ventilations ineffective and intubation difficult to perform.
- Oropharyngeal bleeding can further complicate airway management because the view of the epiglottis and vocal cords is obscured.
- Cricothyrotomy may be indicated if oral endotracheal intubation is impossible.

Complete upper-airway obstruction

- Complete obstruction of the upper airway will prevent effective BVM ventilations as well as the passage of an endotracheal tube between the vocal cords. Common causes of upper-airway obstruction include:
  - Foreign body
  - Epiglottitis
  - Airway burns with swelling
  - Anaphylaxis with laryngeal edema
- Cricothyrotomy may be necessary if attempts to clear the airway using less invasive techniques fail.

Clenched teeth (trismus)

- Trismus is commonly associated with severe head injury as well as mandibular fractures.
- Cricothyrotomy would be indicated only if you are not authorized or able to perform rapid sequence intubation (RSI).

Summary

In the vast majority of cases, the paramedic is able to establish and maintain a patent airway with relative ease. However, some situations can present a challenge to even the most experienced intubator.

Airway management in the patient with severe maxillofacial trauma can be especially difficult. Injuries to the face are commonly associated with mandibular fractures, airway swelling, and oropharyngeal bleeding. Such injuries often prevent effective ventilation with a BVM and can obscure an adequate laryngoscopic view of the vocal cords, making endotracheal intubation extremely difficult, if not impossible.

Dual-lumen airway devices are an acceptable alternative to endotracheal intubation; however, in patients with copious oral secretions or oropharyngeal bleeding, they will not adequately protect the airway from aspiration.

As with any patient, efforts to secure and maintain a patent airway should begin with basic measures. If these fail, you must then take measures to secure the airway with advanced techniques. Endotracheal intubation should be attempted; however, if this fails, a cricothyrotomy, if allowed by locally established protocols, must be performed without delay. Regardless of the patient's condition, the airway must remain patent at all times.

16

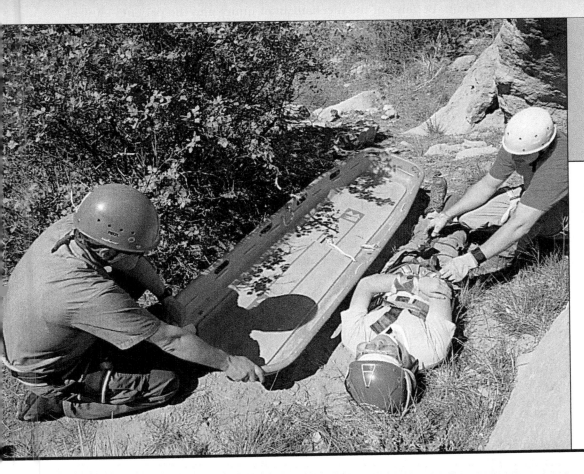

20-Year-Old Male Who Fell from a Cliff

At 2:30 PM, you are dispatched to a nearby state park where a 20-year-old male has fallen from a cliff. High-angle rescuers have delivered the patient to a central staging area, where you will meet them. Your response time to the scene is approximately 15 minutes.

You arrive at the scene at 2:45 PM. Rescue personnel advise you that the patient fell approximately 25 feet from a cliff while hiking. They fully immobilized his spine and then evacuated him to the staging area with a basket stretcher. Your partner opens the trauma kit while you perform an initial assessment **(Table 16-1)**.

Table 16-1 Initial Assessment

Mechanism of Injury	Fall from a significant height
Level of Consciousness	Conscious and alert, restless
Chief Complaint	"I can't feel or move my legs."
Airway and Breathing	Airway is patent; respirations, increased and shallow.
Circulation	Radial pulse is slow, weak, and regular; no gross bleeding noted; skin is warm and dry.

Your partner attempts to provide ventilatory assistance to treat the patient's shallow respirations; however, he will not tolerate the BVM. A nonrebreathing mask is applied and set at 15 L/min. Because of the mechanism of injury and the patient's clinical presentation, you and your partner suspect that this patient is in neurogenic shock.

1. What is the pathophysiology of neurogenic shock?

_____

_____

_____

_____

As your partner prepares to initiate further treatment, you perform a rapid trauma assessment of the patient (Table 16-2). Because the closest trauma center is 1 hour away by ground, you request aeromedical transport. You are advised that the helicopter will arrive at the scene in approximately 15 minutes.

Table 16-2 Rapid Trauma Assessment

Head	Abrasions to the forehead, no major bleeding
Neck	Trachea is midline; jugular veins, normal; no cervical spine deformities.
Chest	Chest wall, stable and symmetrical; breath sounds, clear and equal bilaterally to auscultation
Abdomen/Pelvis	Abdomen, soft and nontender; pelvis, stable
Lower Extremities	Closed deformity to the left mid-shaft femur; pedal pulses, bilaterally absent; the patient cannot feel or move his lower extremities.
Upper Extremities	Numerous abrasions to both arms; radial pulses, weakly present; sensory and motor functions, grossly intact
Posterior	Unable to assess (the patient is on a long spine board); a rescuer tells you that there was swelling and tenderness to the lower thoracic region of the spine.

2. How does the clinical presentation of neurogenic shock differ from that of hypovolemic shock?

_____

_____

_____

_____

The patient is loaded into the ambulance, where you await the arrival of the helicopter. After establishing two large-bore IV lines of normal saline, you attach a cardiac monitor, which reveals a sinus bradycardia at 55 beats per minute. The patient remains conscious while you obtain baseline vital signs and a SAMPLE history (Table 16-3).

Table 16-3 Baseline Vital Signs and SAMPLE History

Blood Pressure	80/50 mm Hg
Pulse	54 beats/min, weak and regular
Respirations	24 breaths/min and shallow
Oxygen Saturation	95% (on 100% oxygen)
Signs and Symptoms	Hypotension, swelling and tenderness to the lower thoracic region of the spine, closed deformity to the left femur
Allergies	None
Medications	None
Pertinent Past History	None
Last Oral Intake	"I ate a sandwich about 2 hours ago."
Events Leading to the Injury	"I was hiking when I lost my footing and fell from a ledge."

3. How is neurogenic shock treated in the prehospital setting?

_____

_____

_____

_____

Further treatment is provided. Because the estimated time of arrival of the helicopter is less than 5 minutes, you do not have time to perform a detailed physical examination. Therefore, you perform a quick ongoing assessment **(Table 16-4)** and prepare the patient for air transport.

Table 16-4 Ongoing Assessment

Level of Consciousness	Conscious and alert to person, place, and time; less restless
Airway and Breathing	Airway remains patent; respirations, 22 breaths/min with adequate tidal volume
Oxygen Saturation	98% (on 100% oxygen)
Blood Pressure	98/58 mm Hg
Pulse	70 beats/min and regular; stronger radial pulses
ECG	Normal sinus rhythm

4. When is it appropriate to transport a trauma patient by air?

_____

_____

_____

_____

The helicopter arrives, and you transfer care of the patient to the flight paramedic. The patient, whose condition has improved, is transported to a trauma center. The patient was diagnosed with a fracture of the tenth thoracic vertebrae and spinal cord swelling. After further stabilization in the emergency department, the patient was taken to the operating room by an orthopaedic surgeon for operative stabilization of his femur and spinal fractures. After surgery, he was admitted to an intensive care unit for further observation. He later recovered partial neurologic function and was transferred to a rehabilitation facility.

1. What is the pathophysiology of neurogenic shock?

Neurogenic shock is caused by an interruption of sympathetic nervous system control between the brain and the rest of the body. Spinal cord injury is the most common cause of neurogenic shock; therefore, it is commonly referred to as *spinal shock*. Other terms are also used to describe neurogenic shock, including *high-space shock* and *vasogenic shock*.

Before discussing the pathophysiology of neurogenic shock, a brief review of normal sympathetic nervous system function is in order.

The sympathetic nervous system regulates heart rate and contractility and blood vessel diameter by releasing catecholamines (epinephrine and norepinephrine) into the bloodstream. These catecholamines, under normal conditions, keep the vascular bed mildly constricted in order to maintain adequate perfusion.

When arterial blood pressure falls, baroreceptors, which are located in the carotid sinus and aortic arch, send messages to the brain via the nervous system. The brain then sends messages via the sympathetic nervous system to the adrenal medulla, causing increased catecholamine production.

Norepinephrine, which stimulates alpha$_1$ receptor sites, causes vasoconstriction and shunting of blood to vital organs of the body. Epinephrine stimulates beta$_1$ and beta$_2$ receptor sites, resulting in an increased heart rate, increased myocardial contractility, and bronchodilation.

The physiologic response of the sympathetic nervous system allows the body to compensate for low cardiac output states, such as shock.

In neurogenic shock, normal sympathetic nervous system function is interrupted; therefore, the normal compensatory response of the body to shock does not occur. Injury to the spinal cord causes dilation of the blood vessels supplied by the spinal nerves distal to the injury, resulting in decreased systemic vascular resistance, hypotension, and loss of body temperature control **(Figure 16-1)**.

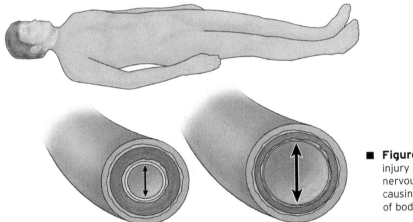

■ **Figure 16-1** Spinal cord injury interrupts sympathetic nervous system function, causing vasodilation and loss of body temperature control.

Although the patient in neurogenic shock has not lost actual blood volume, the normal blood volume (5 to 6 liters) can no longer adequately fill the enlarged vascular space. The patient, therefore, experiences a *relative hypovolemia*.

Because the vascular space is enlarged, systemic venous pooling occurs with a resultant decrease in cardiac preload. Because cardiac preload is reduced, the atria fill inadequately, and their contractions are not sufficient enough to stretch the ventricular walls (Frank-Starling effect). When the ventricular walls stretch inadequately, stroke volume, and thus cardiac output, is reduced.

2. How does the clinical presentation of neurogenic shock differ from that of hypovolemic shock?

Although neurogenic and hypovolemic shock both cause significant hemodynamic compromise, their clinical presentations are distinctly different.

Because neurogenic shock blocks the actions of the sympathetic nervous system, catecholamines are not released into the bloodstream. Therefore, the classic signs of shock (ie, tachycardia, diaphoresis) are absent.

Vasodilation causes the skin to remain pink, warm, and dry below the level of the spinal injury. However, proximal to the injury, where sympathetic nerve fibers remain intact, the skin typically becomes cool, clammy, and pale.

The heart rate, which is classically increased in hypovolemic shock, is slow and weak in patients with neurogenic shock. This is caused by a decrease in circulating epinephrine and the continued, unopposed effects of the parasympathetic nervous system.

Because of catecholamines circulating in the bloodstream prior to the injury, blood pressure is transiently maintained; however, the patient quickly becomes hypotensive because these catecholamines are rapidly depleted.

Unless brainstem injury has occurred, the phrenic nerves are still able to send messages to the respiratory muscles and diaphragm to increase performance; therefore, the patient with neurogenic shock will typically have an increased respiratory rate. If, however, injury to the spinal column occurs in the cervical region, paralysis of the diaphragm, intercostal muscles, or both, may occur.

When compared with hypovolemic shock, the patient in neurogenic shock presents in a significantly different manner **(Table 16-5)**.

Table 16-5 Hypovolemic Shock versus Neurogenic Shock

Assessment	Hypovolemic	Neurogenic
Heart rate	Increased	Slow
Blood pressure	Low	Low
Skin	Cool, pale, and diaphoretic	Pink, warm, and dry
Respirations	Increased	Increased

Because their overall presentation is atypical of hypovolemic shock, patients with neurogenic shock are frequently overlooked, at least initially, in the prehospital setting. This is especially true in multiple-patient incidents that require rapid triage.

Hypovolemic patients, because they are often noticeably diaphoretic and restless, tend to quickly catch the paramedic's eye. However, because the patient in neurogenic shock is usually not diaphoretic, and spinal cord damage with paralysis may prevent them from moving about anxiously, their condition may not be so obvious.

A careful, systematic patient assessment is required to rapidly identify the signs and symptoms of neurogenic shock and begin immediate treatment of the patient. Compared with hypovolemic shock, neurogenic shock is a relatively uncommon occurrence. However, if not recognized and promptly treated, neurogenic shock can result in death by mechanisms similar to other types of shock.

3. How is neurogenic shock treated in the prehospital setting?

The initial prehospital management for patients with neurogenic shock begins by ensuring a patent airway and effective breathing with simultaneous stabilization of the cervical spine. While one partner manages the patient's airway, the other partner should immediately control any severe external bleeding.

Administer 100% supplemental oxygen via nonrebreathing mask if the patient is breathing adequately. If the patient is breathing inadequately, as evidenced by a reduction in tidal volume (shallow breaths) or respirations that are too fast or too slow, assisted ventilations with a BVM device will be necessary.

Because of the severe vasodilation associated with neurogenic shock, the patient is at risk for hypothermia; therefore, apply blankets to maintain body heat. Additionally, any patient in shock should have his or her cardiac rhythm monitored.

Hypotension secondary to neurogenic shock should be treated initially with IV crystalloids. After establishing two large-bore IV lines, infuse normal saline or lactated ringers in 20 mL/kg increments, followed by reassessment of the blood pressure. Repeat fluid boluses as needed or as directed by medical control.

If the patient's blood pressure does not improve with IV fluid boluses, consider administering one of the following vasopressor medications, as authorized by direct medical control or locally established protocols:

- **Dopamine (Intropin)**
  - Dopamine is a naturally occurring catecholamine; varying effects are observed at different doses.
    - At doses of 5 to 10 µg/kg/min, dopamine increases the heart rate and myocardial contractility by stimulating selective $beta_1$ receptor sites.
    - Doses of greater than 10 µk/kg/min cause systemic vasoconstriction by stimulating alpha receptor sites.

- **Norepinephrine (Levophed)**
  - Norepinephrine is also a naturally occurring catecholamine that stimulates both alpha and $beta_1$ receptor sites, causing vasoconstriction and increased myocardial contractility.
    - Dilute 4 mg of norepinephrine in 250 mL of D_5W, yielding a concentration of 16 µg/mL (0.016 mg/mL).
    - Begin the infusion at 0.5 to 1.0 µg/min (up to 30 µg/min) titrated to the desired effect (eg, improved blood pressure and perfusion).

Norepinephrine constricts the renal and mesenteric vasculature, and is therefore used less often than dopamine in the prehospital setting. Consult with medical control or follow locally established protocols regarding pharmacological management for neurogenic shock.

In certain cases, medical control may order you to administer atropine sulfate at a dose of 0.05 mg via IV push. Because bradycardia in neurogenic shock is an effect of unopposed parasympathetic stimulation, atropine, a parasympathetic blocker, may increase the patient's heart rate and improve perfusion.

Consult with medical control regarding the use of the pneumatic antishock garment (PASG) to treat hypotension associated with neurogenic shock. Although the PASG may combat vasodilation in neurogenic shock by increasing systemic vascular resistance, research has yet to demonstrate that the device contributes to a better patient outcome.

Spinal injury, and thus neurogenic shock, can be worsened by the processes of inflammation and swelling in and around the spinal cord. Synthetic glucocorticoids (steroids) such as methylprednisolone (Solu-Medrol) or dexamethasone (Decadron, Hexadrol) may be administered to reduce inflammation and swelling. Steroids, especially Solu-Medrol, are very effective in decreasing the severity of spinal cord injury, especially if administered within the first 8 hours following the injury.

Further prehospital management for neurogenic shock includes full spinal immobilization, prompt transport to a trauma center, and continuous monitoring.

4. When is it appropriate to transport a trauma patient by air?

A number of factors should be considered when determining the most appropriate mode of transport for the trauma patient. Although criteria to assist the paramedic in making the appropriate transport mode decision vary in each EMS system, it is generally agreed upon that the patient should be transported by ground if a trauma center can be reached within 60 minutes following the injury (ie, the golden hour). The paramedic should, however, consult with medical control or follow locally established protocols regarding the use of aeromedical transportation.

In the prehospital setting, helicopters are most commonly used to evacuate critical trauma patients to the appropriate facility. Fixed-wing aircraft, because they need a more controlled landing environment (ie, a runway), are clearly not practical. A helicopter landing zone (LZ) need only be 100 by 100 feet and free of obstructions and power lines.

Although most emergency procedures provided by flight paramedics can be provided by ground transport paramedics, the use of helicopters is especially beneficial because of their rapid response time both to the scene and from the scene to a trauma center.

When determining the most appropriate mode of transport, the paramedic should quickly answer the following questions:

■ Will the time required for ground transport pose a threat to the patient's survival and recovery?

■ Are there any weather, road, or traffic conditions that would unnecessarily delay ground transport and the patient's access to definitive care?

■ Are critical care personnel (eg, critical care paramedics or nurses) and/or specialized equipment required to more effectively care for the patient during transport?

When en route to an emergency scene involving a critically injured patient, you should consider both the advantages and disadvantages of using aeromedical transport services (Table 16-6).

If you are unsure if aeromedical transport will be needed, it is not unreasonable to notify the dispatcher and have them place the aircraft on standby. This way, if the decision is made to evacuate the patient by air, unnecessary delays will be avoided. If, after rapidly assessing the patient, you determine that ground transport is more appropriate, you can always cancel, or stand down, the aircraft.

Be certain to understand your local protocols regarding helicopter availability and stand-by requirements. Air transport decisions should always be based on the best interests of the patient, not the convenience of the paramedic.

Table 16-6 Advantages and Disadvantages of Aeromedical Transport

Advantages
- Rapid response times to and from the scene
  - Quicker access to definitive care
- Geographic barriers (eg, mountainous terrain) can be avoided
- Frees up ground ambulances to respond to other calls
- Helicopters can fly even if road conditions are unfavorable.
- In rural areas, where BLS care is exclusive, the level of care provided may be upgraded.
- Safer for the patient
  - Helicopter crashes are less common than ambulance crashes.

Disadvantages
- In urban settings, within 30 miles of the hospital, ground transport is usually faster.
- Inclement weather (eg, fog, lightning) may prevent the aircraft from flying.
- Aeromedical transport is far more costly than ground transport.
- The helicopter, if it is the only one available, will be unable to respond to other calls.
- Noise in the aircraft may prevent effective communication with the patient.
- Helicopters have space and weight limitations.

Summary

Neurogenic shock causes hemodynamic compromise by impairing the sympathetic nervous system and preventing the release of catecholamines. Spinal injury is the most common cause of neurogenic shock, which should be suspected when a patient presents with hypotension but doesn't have other classic signs of shock (ie, tachycardia, diaphoresis).

Because no catecholamines are released in neurogenic shock, a reflex vasodilation occurs. This enlarges the vascular space, creating a *relative hypovolemia* that leads to hypoperfusion of the vital organs of the body. Unopposed parasympathetic function causes the heart rate to become slow and weak, instead of the typical tachycardia seen in other types of shock where the sympathetic nervous system is intact.

The paramedic must perform a careful, systematic patient assessment and recognize the typical clinical presentation of neurogenic shock. As with any other type of shock, neurogenic shock can be fatal.

Prehospital management for the patient in neurogenic shock includes ensuring airway patency, effective breathing, and effective circulation. Administer 100% oxygen by nonrebreathing mask or, if the patient is breathing inadequately, assisted ventilations with a BVM device. Simultaneous stabilization and immobilization of the patient's spine is critical, because concomitant spinal injury frequently accompanies neurogenic shock.

Further management includes providing blankets to limit body heat loss and IV crystalloid boluses to support blood pressure. Vasopressor therapy (eg, dopamine, norepinephrine) may be needed if IV fluids are unsuccessful in maintaining blood pressure.

Medical control may order the administration of steroids, such as Solu-Medrol or Decadron, to reduce inflammation and swelling in and around the spinal cord.

As with any critical trauma patient, rapid transport to a trauma center is vital so that definitive care can be initiated as soon as possible. The use of aeromedical transportation can facilitate this process.

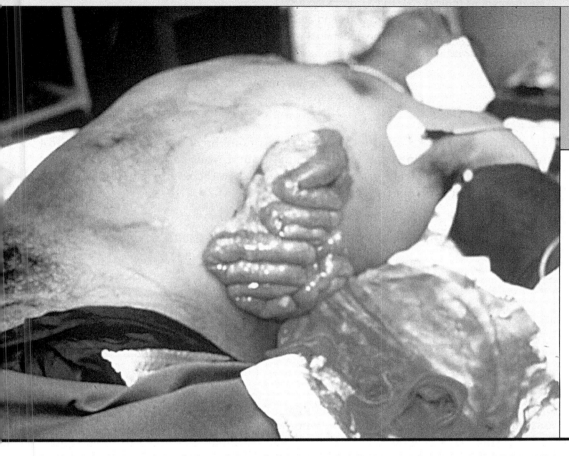

17

44-Year-Old Male with an Open Abdominal Wound

At 4:45 PM, you are dispatched to a furniture manufacturing plant where a 44-year-old male who was involved in a table saw accident has sustained an open abdominal wound. Your response time to the scene is approximately 8 minutes.

You arrive at the scene at 5:03 PM, where you are met by the patient's supervisor. The supervisor tells you that the patient slipped and fell across the blade of a table saw. As you approach the patient, you can see that he is conscious, restless, and has a large abdominal evisceration. You immediately direct your partner to care for the open abdominal wound while you perform an initial assessment of the patient (Table 17-1).

1. What complications are associated with an abdominal evisceration?

_____

_____

_____

_____

Table 17-1 Initial Assessment

Mechanism of Injury	Fell across a table saw
Level of Consciousness	Conscious and alert, extremely restless
Chief Complaint	Open abdominal wound
Airway and Breathing	Airway is patent; respirations, increased with adequate tidal volume.
Circulation	Radial pulse, weak and rapid; skin is pale, cool, and clammy; bleeding from a large abdominal evisceration (controlled); no other gross bleeding.

You administer 100% oxygen to the patient via a nonrebreathing mask. After controlling the external bleeding from the abdominal wound, your partner covers the wound with dressings and bandages. A police officer arrives at the scene, and you ask him to retrieve the stretcher from the ambulance.

2. What is the appropriate care for an abdominal evisceration?

_____

_____

_____

_____

After appropriately caring for the abdominal wound, you perform a rapid trauma assessment **(Table 17-2)** on the patient, who remains conscious and alert, but restless. You and your partner agree that IV therapy will be initiated en route to the hospital.

Table 17-2 Rapid Trauma Assessment

Head	No obvious trauma
Neck	Trachea is midline; jugular veins, normal; no cervical spine deformities.
Chest	No obvious trauma; chest wall, stable and symmetrical; breath sounds, clear and equal bilaterally to auscultation
Abdomen/Pelvis	Large abdominal evisceration (dressed and bandaged); portions of the abdomen adjacent to the evisceration are rigid; pelvis is stable.
Lower Extremities	No obvious trauma; pedal pulses, present; sensory and motor functions, grossly intact
Upper Extremities	No obvious trauma; radial pulses, present; sensory and motor functions, grossly intact
Posterior	No obvious trauma

The patient is placed onto the stretcher and quickly loaded into the ambulance. After obtaining baseline vital signs and a SAMPLE history **(Table 17-3)**, you proceed to the nearest trauma center, which is approximately 15 miles away. En route, you prepare to initiate IV therapy.

Table 17-3 Baseline Vital Signs and SAMPLE History

Blood Pressure	114/60 mm Hg
Pulse	120 beats/min, weak and regular
Respirations	22 breaths/min, adequate tidal volume
Oxygen Saturation	98% (on 100% oxygen)
Signs and Symptoms	Large abdominal evisceration, signs of shock
Allergies	None
Medications	Lipitor
Pertinent Past History	High cholesterol
Last Oral Intake	"I ate lunch about 3 hours ago."
Events Leading to the Injury	"I was cutting a 2 × 4 in half, when I slipped and fell across the blade of the table saw."

3. What is the appropriate IV fluid regimen for this patient?

_____

_____

_____

_____

You have established two large-bore IV lines of normal saline and have set them to the appropriate flow rate. The patient remains conscious and alert, but restless. A cardiac monitor is applied and reveals a sinus tachycardia at 120 beats/min. With an estimated time of arrival at the trauma center of 10 minutes, you perform a detailed physical examination on the patient **(Table 17-4)**.

Table 17-4 Detailed Physical Examination

Head and Face	No obvious trauma to the scalp; ears, nose, and mouth are clear; pupils are midpoint, equal, and reactive to light.
Neck	Trachea is midline; jugular veins, normal, no cervical spine deformities.
Chest	No obvious trauma; chest wall, stable and symmetrical; breath sounds, clear and equal bilaterally to auscultation
Abdomen/Pelvis	Large abdominal evisceration (dressed and bandaged); abdomen adjacent to the evisceration is rigid; pelvis is stable.
Lower Extremities	No obvious trauma; pedal pulses, present; sensory and motor functions, grossly intact
Upper Extremities	No obvious trauma, radial pulses, present; sensory and motor functions, grossly intact
Posterior	No obvious trauma

Because of the patient's abdominal rigidity, you suspect intraabdominal bleeding. You reassess the patient and note that his blood pressure is now 80/50 mm Hg and his pulse is 130 beats/min. Additionally, the patient is becoming more restless. You adjust your IV flow rates accordingly to maintain adequate perfusion.

4. What major solid organs lie in the true abdomen? What are their functions?

_____

_____

_____

_____

The patient's blood pressure is stabilized with IV fluids. With an estimated time of arrival at the trauma center of 5 minutes, you perform an ongoing assessment (Table 17-5) and then call your radio report to the receiving facility.

Table 17-5 Ongoing Assessment

Level of Consciousness	Conscious and alert, restless
Airway and Breathing	Airway remains patent; respirations, 22 breaths/min with adequate tidal volume
Oxygen Saturation	98% (on 100% oxygen)
Blood Pressure	96/56 mm Hg
Pulse	110 beats/min, regular and stronger
ECG	Sinus tachycardia

The patient is delivered to the emergency department, and you give your verbal report to the attending physician. Following initial stabilization in the emergency department, which includes blood administration, the patient is taken immediately to surgery, where his evisceration and a splenic laceration were both repaired. He was admitted to the surgical intensive care unit and eventually recovered.

1. What complications are associated with an abdominal evisceration?

An abdominal evisceration most commonly occurs through the anterior abdominal wall. It usually involves protrusion of the small intestine and/or omentum (a fold of peritoneum that connects or supports the abdominal structures).

As with any open abdominal wound, the immediate risk to the patient's life is external hemorrhage, which must be controlled immediately. If, however, other internal abdominal organs or structures are injured as well (eg, liver, spleen), intraabdominal hemorrhage, which cannot be controlled in the prehospital setting, may also be present.

Infarction and necrosis of the bowel or omentum can occur if circulation to the exposed viscera is compromised. Additionally, because open abdominal wounds can result in a significant loss of body heat, the patient is at risk for hypothermia.

If the exposed bowel is lacerated, spillage of intestinal contents can occur, resulting in peritonitis and life-threatening sepsis. Although this is a complication likely to be encountered later, it affects how you will care for the eviscerated bowel in the prehospital setting (ie, preventing contamination of the exposed bowel).

2. What is the appropriate care for an abdominal evisceration?

The goals of managing an abdominal evisceration are to control external bleeding and prevent contamination of the exposed bowel. First and foremost, you must control any external hemorrhage with direct pressure. However, because you do not want to push the protruding bowel back into the abdominal cavity, you should apply just enough pressure to effectively control the bleeding.

Because bacteria can be introduced into the peritoneal space, you should never attempt to replace the protruding bowel back into the abdominal cavity. If the bowel is lacerated, there is an additional risk of content spillage into the peritoneum, which may result in peritonitis and life-threatening sepsis.

The open abdomen radiates body heat very effectively, and the exposed bowel can rapidly lose fluid. Therefore, the exposed viscera must be kept warm and moist. After controlling external bleeding, the evisceration should be covered with a moist sterile dressing (eg, multitrauma dressing), which should be secured in place with a dry sterile dressing **(Figure 17-1)**. To retain moisture and to minimize contamination of the exposed bowel, an occlusive dressing can be placed in between the moist and dry dressings. To provide further support and protection for the protruding bowel, you can apply padding in a circumferential manner, so as to "corral" the exposed bowel.

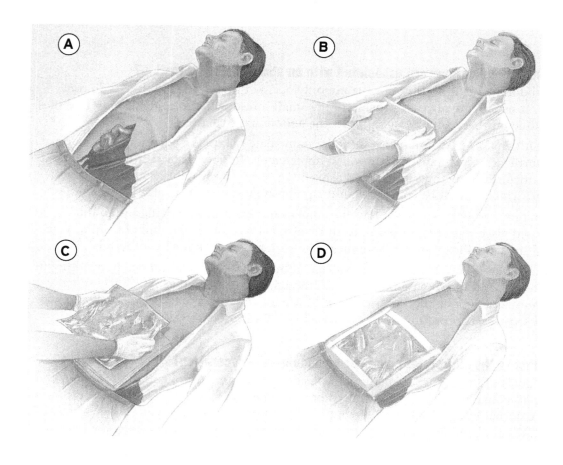

■ **Figure 17-1** (A.) The open abdomen radiates body heat rapidly and must be covered. (B.) Cover the wound with a moist sterile dressing. Consider placing an occlusive dressing over the moist dressing. (C.) Cover the moist dressing with a dry sterile dressing. (D.) Secure the dressings in place with tape.

Never touch or handle the exposed bowel with your bare hands, because this only increases the risk of infection and further injury. Some EMS systems advocate placing aluminum foil over the exposed bowel to help retain body heat; however, this may increase the risk of lacerating the bowel. When covering the bowel, avoid the use of material that is adherent or loses its substance when wet. Such materials include toilet or tissue paper, paper towels, and absorbent cotton.

Use of the pneumatic antishock garment (PASG) is contraindicated in the management of an abdominal evisceration or any open abdominal wound. Clearly, inflation of the abdominal compartment of the PASG would force the protruding bowel back into the abdominal cavity. Additionally, inflation of the leg compartments may exacerbate external and internal hemorrhage as blood is forced from the lower extremities.

3. What is the appropriate IV fluid regimen for this patient?

This patient is clearly demonstrating signs of shock (ie, restlessness, diaphoresis, tachycardia); however, his blood pressure of 114/60 mm Hg suggests that he is in compensated shock, at least for the time being.

Decompensated shock is typically marked by a fall in the patient's blood pressure and indicates that the body is no longer able to effectively compensate for hypoperfusion.

For the patient in shock, IV crystalloid fluids (eg, normal saline, lactated ringers) should be administered to maintain a systolic blood pressure of at least 90 mm Hg. Although the blood pressure needed to maintain adequate perfusion varies in each person, a systolic blood pressure of at least 90 mm Hg will usually maintain adequate perfusion in the average 70-kg adult.

For this patient, two large-bore IV lines of normal saline or lactated ringers should be initiated. However, because his blood pressure is maintained at an acceptable level, the flow rate of the IVs should be set to keep the vein open. Carefully monitor the patient's blood pressure as well as other indicators of perfusion (eg, mental status, peripheral pulses) and be prepared to infuse the IV fluids as needed to maintain adequate perfusion.

The goal of IV therapy for the patient in shock is to maintain the systolic blood pressure, not rapidly increase it. This is especially true in patients with suspected internal bleeding, such as your patient, whose rigid abdomen suggests intraabdominal hemorrhage.

Following injury to the internal vasculature and organs, a predictable series of events takes place that result in hemostasis (natural cessation of bleeding). During hemostasis, chemicals released from the vessel wall cause local vasoconstriction and platelet activation, resulting in the formation of a temporary "plug." Additionally, tissue thromboplastin activates a cascade of events that leads to the formation of thrombin, a chemical that promotes the conversion of fibrinogen to fibrin. Fibrin binds to the temporary platelet plug, forming the final mature clot **(Figure 17-2)**.

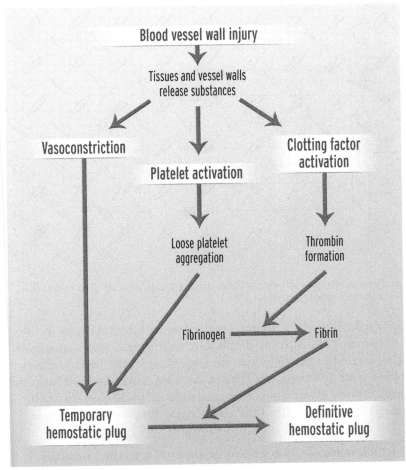

■ **Figure 17-2** Hemostasis is the body's natural ability to spontaneously stop bleeding through local vasoconstriction and the formation of a platelet plug.

Rapid IV fluid infusion could cause a sudden increase in the patient's blood pressure, thus causing the platelet plug, formed by hemostasis, to rupture. This would exacerbate internal bleeding, resulting in deterioration of the patient's condition. Remember, internal bleeding requires surgical intervention and cannot be controlled in the prehospital setting.

If, however, the patient's blood pressure begins to fall, infuse normal saline or lactated ringers in 20 mL/kg increments and then reassess the blood pressure. If needed, infuse additional IV fluids to maintain a systolic blood pressure of at least 90 mm Hg.

4. What major solid organs lie in the true abdomen? What are their functions?

Because abdominal eviscerations are most commonly caused by penetrating trauma, organs within the true abdomen are commonly injured. The true abdomen, also referred to as the anterior abdomen, contains two major solid organs: the liver and the spleen **(Figure 17-3)**. The pancreas and kidneys, which are also major solid organs, lie in the retroperitoneal space, which is located behind the true abdomen.

Hollow organs (eg, stomach, intestines), when injured, spill their contents into the abdominal cavity, causing peritonitis and infection. Solid organs, however, bleed profusely when crushed or penetrated. This is especially true of the liver and the spleen, which are both highly vascular organs.

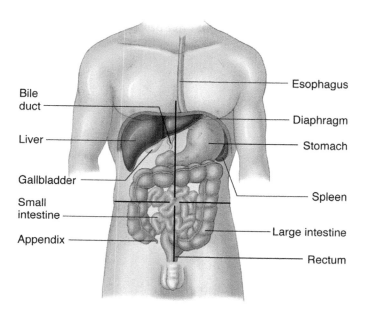

■ **Figure 17-3** The liver and spleen, which lie in the true abdomen, are highly vascular solid organs that bleed profusely when crushed or penetrated.

The liver, which weighs approximately 3 pounds, is the largest internal organ in the human body. The liver is located beneath the diaphragm in the right upper quadrant of the abdomen. Blood is carried to the liver via two large vessels: the hepatic artery (carries oxygen-rich blood from the aorta) and the portal vein (directs blood from the intestines for processing). At any given time, approximately 20 to 30 percent of the total body blood volume is contained within the liver. Major functions of the liver include the following:

■ **Production of bile,** which is necessary for the digestion of fat in the intestines

- **Manufacture of the following essential blood components:**
  - Fibrinogen and other clotting factors that are necessary for the coagulation process
    - Injury to the liver can severely impair the body's hemostatic processes.
  - Albumin, which is needed for intracellular fluid balance
  - Immunoglobulins, which are key components of the immune response
- **Production and storage of glucose in the form of glycogen**
  - The liver stores glucose in the form of glycogen and breaks it down into glucose when the body needs it for energy.
- **Detoxification of harmful substances from the blood,** such as alcohol and drugs
  - Phagocytic cells in the liver, called Kupffer cells, remove foreign particles from the blood.
- **Storage of important vitamins and minerals,** including vitamins A, D, K, and B_{12}

The spleen, which is located behind the stomach in the left upper abdominal quadrant, acts as a filter against foreign organisms that infect the bloodstream and also filters out and breaks down old red blood cells from the bloodstream. These splenic functions are performed by phagocytic cells that are capable of engulfing and destroying bacteria, parasites, and other organisms.

Ordinarily, the spleen manufactures red blood cells only toward the end of fetal life. Following birth, that function is assumed by the bone marrow. However, in cases of bone marrow breakdown, the spleen can revert back to its fetal function.

The spleen also acts as a blood reservoir. During stress or at other times when additional blood is needed, the spleen contracts, forcing stored blood into the systemic circulation.

Summary

Penetrating abdominal trauma frequently results in the death of the trauma patient. Injuries such as stabbings, large lacerations, and gunshot wounds can result in abdominal eviscerations, in which a portion of the bowel protrudes through the abdominal wall.

Open abdominal injuries result in rapid loss of body heat. If the abdominal injury is large, hypothermia may occur. Additionally, the exposed bowel loses fluid rapidly and may dry. If the exposed bowel is lacerated, spillage of its contents may occur, resulting in peritonitis and infection. If circulation to the exposed bowel is compromised, infarction and necrosis of the bowel may occur.

Injury to the internal abdominal organs, such as the liver and spleen, may also be present with an abdominal evisceration. Bleeding from these highly vascular organs can be profuse, causing severe hemodynamic compromise and shock.

After ensuring a patent airway and adequate ventilation, emergency care for the patient with an abdominal evisceration includes treatment for shock: 100% supplemental oxygen, thermal management, and IV fluids as needed to maintain adequate perfusion. Management of critically injured patients should include cardiac rhythm and oxygen saturation monitoring if possible. Care for the eviscerated bowel itself involves covering the bowel with a moist sterile dressing. The moist dressing is then covered with a dry sterile dressing. Under no circumstances should you touch the exposed bowel with your bare hands or attempt to place it back into the abdominal cavity.

Rapidly transport the patient to a trauma center, with close continuous monitoring of the patient en route. Notify the receiving facility early so that the appropriate hospital resources (eg, the trauma team, surgery) are available.

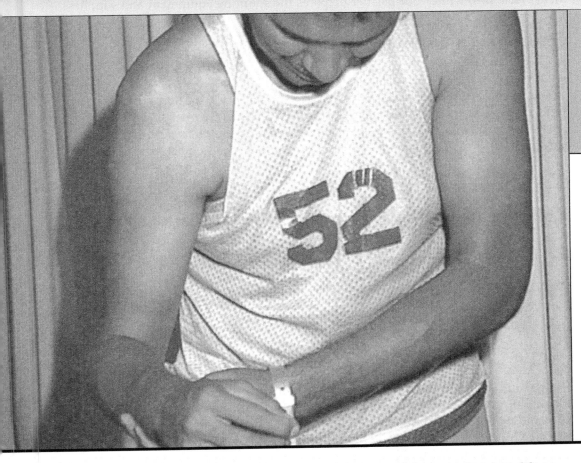

18

20-Year-Old Male with a Shoulder Injury

At 2:25 PM, you are dispatched to a local gym where a 20-year-old male has injured his shoulder while playing basketball. Your response time to the scene is approximately 7 minutes.

You arrive at the scene at 2:32 PM and are escorted to the patient by a fellow team-mate. You find the patient leaning forward, supporting his right arm. There is a noticeable anterior bulge of his upper right arm.

1. What specific injury has this patient most likely sustained?

_____

_____

_____

_____

The patient tells you that he fell against his outstretched arm while playing basketball. He denies loss of consciousness or any other injuries. You perform an initial assessment (Table 18-1) while your partner prepares the splinting equipment and supplies.

Table 18-1 Initial Assessment

Mechanism of Injury	Fell on an outstretched arm
Level of Consciousness	Conscious and alert to person, place, and time
Chief Complaint	"My right shoulder hurts and I can't move my arm."
Airway and Breathing	Airway is patent; respirations, normal rate and depth.
Circulation	Pulse is increased, strong, and regular; skin is pink, warm, and moist; no bleeding is present.

2. What signs and symptoms are commonly associated with this patient's injury?

_____

_____

_____

While your partner prepares to splint the patient's shoulder and arm, you perform a focused physical examination (Table 18-2). The patient continues to complain of severe pain and will not allow you to move his arm. He asks if there is something that you can give him for the pain.

Table 18-2 Focused Physical Examination

Inspection	Anterior bulge of the right upper arm, shoulder appears flattened
Palpation	Skin distal to the injury site is pink, warm, and dry; severe pain is present upon palpation and with any motion of the arm.
Distal Neurovascular Function	Radial pulse, present and strong; capillary refill time, less than 2 seconds; sensory and motor functions, grossly intact

3. What is the appropriate method for immobilizing this patient's injury?

_____

_____

_____

_____

Your partner has appropriately immobilized the patient's arm and shoulder. Distal pulse and motor and sensory functions remain grossly intact following splinting. Out of embarrassment, the patient refuses to be "carried off on a stretcher." On his own accord, he walks to the ambulance. Shortly before departing the scene, you obtain baseline vital signs and a SAMPLE history **(Table 18-3)**.

Table 18-3 Baseline Vital Signs and SAMPLE History

Blood Pressure	118/66 mm Hg
Pulse	100 beats/min, strong and regular
Respirations	18 breaths/min, adequate tidal volume
Oxygen Saturation	99% (on room air)
Signs and Symptoms	Anterior bulge of the right shoulder, severe pain
Allergies	None
Medications	None
Pertinent Past History	None
Last Oral Intake	Lunch, approximately 3 hours ago
Events Leading to the Injury	"I was playing basketball when I tripped over another player and fell."

You begin transport to a community hospital located 20 miles away. En route, the patient continues to complain of severe pain. He remains conscious and alert to person, place, and time. Again, he asks you for something for the pain.

4. What would be appropriate analgesia for this patient?

\
\
\
\

You administer the appropriate pharmacologic agent to the patient, after which he expresses some relief from the pain. You reassess distal pulse and sensory and motor functions in the injured extremity and note that they remain grossly intact. With an estimated time of arrival at the hospital of 10 minutes, you perform an ongoing assessment **(Table 18-4)** and then call your radio report to the receiving facility.

Table 18-4 Ongoing Assessment

Level of Consciousness	Conscious and alert to person, place, and time
Airway and Breathing	Airway remains patent; respirations, 14 breaths/min with adequate tidal volume
Oxygen Saturation	99% (on room air)
Blood Pressure	116/64 mm Hg
Pulse	88 beats/min, strong and regular

The patient is delivered to the emergency department, and you give your verbal report to the charge nurse. Radiographic evaluation reveals an anterior dislocation of the patient's shoulder. After sedating the patient and administering further analgesia, the physician reduces the dislocation with manual traction. He is observed in the emergency department for several hours and then driven home by a friend.

1. What specific injury has this patient most likely sustained?

The anterior bulge that you see to the upper right arm is the proximal portion of the patient's humerus. This type of deformity is consistent with an anterior dislocation of the shoulder. The glenohumeral joint (shoulder joint), a ball-and-socket joint, is where the head of the humerus articulates with the glenoid fossa of the scapula **(Figure 18-1)**.

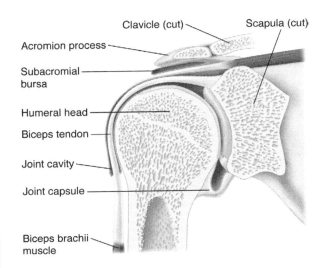

Clavicle (cut)

Scapula (cut)

Acromion process

Subacromial bursa

Humeral head

Biceps tendon

Joint cavity

Joint capsule

Biceps brachii muscle

■ **Figure 18-1** The humeral head articulates with the glenoid fossa of the scapula to form the glenohumeral joint.

The glenohumeral joint is the most frequently dislocated large joint in the body, accounting for over 50 percent of major joint dislocations. Approximately 95 percent of shoulder dislocations are anterior.

Shoulder dislocations occur when trauma to the ligaments of the glenohumeral joint allows the humeral head to separate from the glenoid fossa. Although direct trauma to the shoulder can result in a dislocation, the majority of shoulder dislocations occur when indirect force is applied to the glenohumeral joint after the patient falls on an outstretched arm. This mechanism is common in young patients participating in athletic events or elderly patients who trip and fall.

The glenohumeral joint allows for a broad range of motion; however, because the glenoid fossa is relatively shallow, it is inherently unstable. The subscapularis tendon of the rotator cuff and the superior and inferior glenohumeral ligaments prevent anterior dislocation of the humeral head. When the patient falls on an outstretched arm, the superior acromion process limits abduction and external rotation of the humerus. This forces the head of the humerus out of the glenoid fossa, against the inferior glenohumeral ligament. If the force is sufficient, anterior dislocation of the shoulder occurs **(Figure 18-2)**.

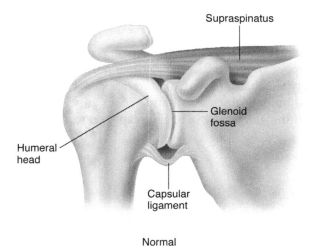

Supraspinatus

Humeral head

Glenoid fossa

Capsular ligament

Normal

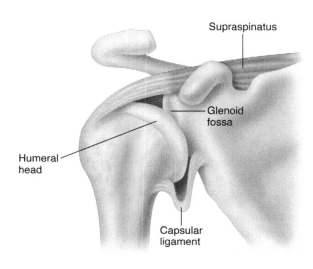

Supraspinatus

Humeral head

Glenoid fossa

Capsular ligament

Anterior dislocation

■ **Figure 18-2** Anterior-inferior dislocation of the shoulder.

2. What signs and symptoms are commonly associated with this patient's injury?

The patient with an anterior shoulder dislocation presents with severe pain and with the affected arm abducted and externally rotated. The patient will typically guard the shoulder and attempt to protect it by holding the dislocated arm in a fixed position away from the chest wall.

The patient will generally have an absence of normal shoulder contour (appears squared off or flattened) and will be unable to move the shoulder joint. The humeral head will typically protrude anteriorly underneath the pectoralis major on the anterior chest wall **(Figure 18-3)**.

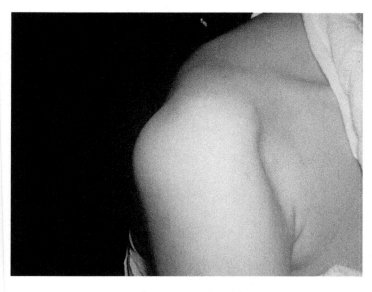

■ **Figure 18-3** In anterior shoulder dislocation, the humeral head protrudes anteriorly, and the shoulder will appear squared off or flattened.

In up to 10 percent of anterior shoulder dislocations, neurologic compromise occurs. The shoulder joint is rich in nerves and vasculature, including the brachial plexus, axillary nerve and artery, and radial nerve.

If the axillary nerve is compromised, the patient may experience numbness to the lateral aspect of the shoulder. Disruption of other nervous structures is far less common. The signs and symptoms of an anterior shoulder dislocation are summarized in **Table 18-5**.

Table 18-5 Signs and Symptoms of Anterior Shoulder Dislocation

Severe pain
Affected arm is abducted and externally rotated.
Abnormal shoulder contour • Squared off or flattened appearance
Parasthesia if nerves and blood vessels are compromised. • Neurologic compromise (typically axillary nerve injury) occurs in up to 10 percent of anterior shoulder dislocations.

3. What is the appropriate method for immobilizing this patient's injury?

Although there are several correct methods for immobilizing a dislocated shoulder, the goal is the same: effectively immobilizing the shoulder without causing further injury.

Because any attempt to bring the arm toward the body will cause the patient severe pain, shoulder dislocations can be difficult to immobilize. The joint must be splinted in a position that is most comfortable for the patient **(Figure 18-4)**.

Pillows or rolled towels can be placed in between the arm and chest for support. When the arm is stabilized in this fashion, the elbow can usually be flexed to 90° without causing further pain.

After positioning padding in between the arm and chest, apply a sling to the forearm and wrist to support the weight of the arm. The entire arm is then secured to the body with a swathe.

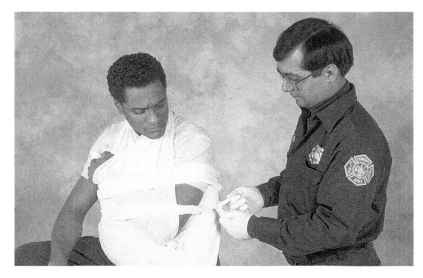

■ Figure 18-4
Splint the joint in a position of comfort and place a pillow or rolled towels between the arm and chest. Apply a sling to the forearm and wrist and then secure the entire arm to the body with a swathe.

Do not hurriedly immobilize a shoulder dislocation. Doing so will only cause the patient unnecessary pain and potentially result in further injury. After properly immobilizing the injury, allow the patient to assume a comfortable position.

4. What would be appropriate analgesia for this patient?

Narcotic analgesics are typically used to relieve the pain associated with isolated orthopedic injuries. Clearly, it would be inappropriate to administer narcotic medications to clinically unstable patients, such as those who are in shock due to multiple fractures. The following narcotic medications are commonly used for pain relief:

- **Morphine sulfate** (Duramorph, Astromorph)
  - IV administration
    - 2 to 4 mg via slow IV push over 1 to 5 minutes
    - May repeat in 5 to 30 minutes to a maximum dose of 10 mg
    - IM or SC administration
    - 5 to 20 mg per 70 kg of body weight
- **Nalbuphine hydrochloride** (Nubain)
  - 10 mg per 70 kg of body weight
    - Can be administered via IV, IM, or SC
- **Meperidine hydrochloride** (Demerol)
  - 15 to 35 mg via IV administration
  - 50 to 100 mg via IM injection

Remember that narcotic medications, including some synthetic narcotics (eg, Nubain), cause CNS depression. Observe the patient for signs of CNS depression, which include hypoventilation, bradycardia, and hypotension. If needed, administer naloxone (Narcan) 0.4 to 2.0 mg via IV or IM administration to counteract the CNS depressant effects.

Summary

The shoulder (glenohumeral joint) is the most frequently dislocated large joint in the body. Nearly 95 percent of all shoulder dislocations occur anteriorly. Although direct trauma to the shoulder can result in dislocation, the most common cause is indirect trauma to the shoulder, such as when the patient falls on an outstretched arm.

The clinical presentation of the patient with an anterior shoulder dislocation includes an anterior bulge of the humeral head and an abnormal contour of the shoulder, which commonly appears flattened or squared off. The shoulder is typically abducted and externally rotated, with the patient guarding the shoulder and holding the affected arm away from the chest wall. Any attempts to move the patient's arm will result in severe pain, and should thus be avoided. Neurologic compromise occurs in approximately 10 percent of patients with anterior shoulder dislocations.

Appropriate care for an anterior shoulder dislocation includes assessing distal circulation and motor and sensory functions, properly splinting the shoulder and arm to allow for a comfortable patient position and to prevent further injury, and then reassessing distal circulation and motor and sensory functions after splinting.

Narcotic analgesic medications (eg, Morphine, Nubain, Demerol) can be administered to the patient for pain relief. As with the administration of narcotic analgesics to any patient, CNS depression may occur, thus requiring the administration of naloxone.

19

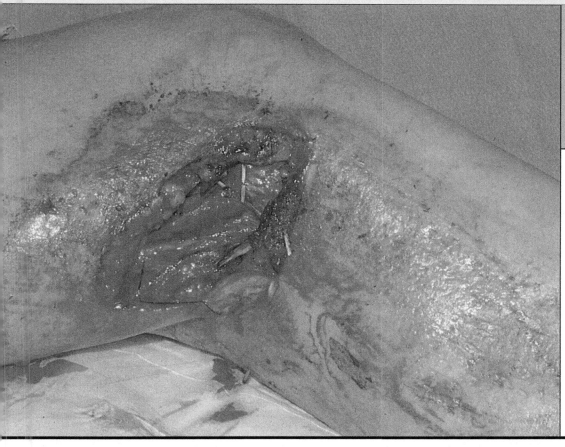

50-Year-Old Male with Severe External Bleeding

You are dispatched to a residence at 325 West San Saba for a 50-year-old male involved in a chainsaw accident. Dispatch advises you that the caller was panicked, stating that the patient was "bleeding to death." The time of call is 9:30 AM, and your response time to the scene is less than 3 minutes.

You arrive at the scene to find the patient sitting in his front yard. He is screaming in pain while attempting to stop the bleeding from a severe avulsion injury behind his right knee. The patient's wife tells you that her husband was cutting wood with a chainsaw. Evidently, the chainsaw slipped and swung around behind him, striking him behind the knee. You perform an initial assessment **(Table 19-1)** while your partner begins immediate treatment.

Table 19-1 Initial Assessment

Mechanism of Injury	Chainsaw injury to the leg
Level of Consciousness	Conscious and alert, restless
Chief Complaint	Severe avulsion injury behind the right knee
Airway and Breathing	Airway is patent; respirations, increased with adequate tidal volume.
Circulation	Pulse is weak and rapid; skin is cool, clammy, and pale; bright red blood is spurting from the injury behind his knee.

1. What is the appropriate order of initial management for this patient?

_____

_____

_____

The appropriate initial management has been provided for the patient. Because the patient is experiencing signs of shock, you perform a rapid trauma assessment **(Table 19-2)**. Your partner quickly retrieves the stretcher from the ambulance.

Table 19-2 Rapid Trauma Assessment

Head	No obvious trauma
Neck	Trachea is midline; jugular veins, normal; no cervical spine deformities.
Chest	No obvious trauma; chest wall, stable and symmetrical; breath sounds, clear and equal bilaterally to auscultation
Abdomen/Pelvis	Abdomen, soft and nontender; pelvis, stable
Lower Extremities	Large avulsion behind right knee (bandaged); pedal pulses, bilaterally absent; sensory and motor functions, grossly intact
Upper Extremities	No obvious trauma; radial pulses, present and weak; sensory and motor functions; grossly intact
Posterior	No obvious trauma

After placing the patient onto the stretcher, he is quickly loaded into the ambulance. While you are setting up your IV lines, your partner notices that blood is soaking through the dressing covering the patient's wound.

2. How will you manage the continued bleeding from the patient's injury?

_____

_____

_____

Additional measures have controlled the bleeding from the patient's injury. While you are preparing to start two large-bore IV lines, your partner obtains baseline vital signs and a SAMPLE history **(Table 19-3)**. A cardiac monitor is applied and reveals a sinus tachycardia at 130 beats per minute.

Table 19-3 Baseline Vital Signs and SAMPLE History

Blood Pressure	84/54 mm Hg
Pulse	132 beats/min, weak and regular
Respirations	24 breaths/min, adequate tidal volume
Oxygen Saturation	96% (on 100% oxygen)
Signs and Symptoms	Avulsion injury with severe bleeding (controlled), signs of shock
Allergies	Demerol, Amoxicillin
Medications	Lotrel
Pertinent Past History	Hypertension
Last Oral Intake	Breakfast, 3 hours ago
Events Leading to the Injury	"I was cutting wood with a chainsaw, when it slipped."

You depart the scene for a trauma center located approximately 25 miles away. Two large-bore IV lines have been successfully established, and you adjust the flow rates accordingly. The patient remains conscious; however, he is increasingly restless.

3. What is the appropriate IV fluid resuscitation regimen for this patient?

_____

_____

_____

_____

4. What is the difference between crystalloid and colloid solutions?

_____

_____

_____

_____

After infusing the appropriate volume of normal saline, the patient's condition has improved. He is less restless, and his blood pressure is now 96/60 mm Hg. After reassessing the bandaged wound and noting that the bleeding remains controlled, you perform a detailed physical examination **(Table 19-4)**.

Table 19-4 Detailed Physical Examination

Head and Face	No obvious trauma to the scalp; ears, nose, and mouth are clear; pupils are midpoint, equal, and reactive to light.
Neck	Trachea is midline; jugular veins, normal; no cervical spine deformities.
Chest	No obvious trauma; chest wall, stable and symmetrical; breath sounds, clear and equal bilaterally to auscultation
Abdomen/Pelvis	Abdomen, soft and nontender; pelvis, stable
Lower Extremities	Large avulsion behind right knee (bandaged); pedal pulses, bilaterally absent; sensory and motor functions, grossly intact
Upper Extremities	No obvious trauma; radial pulses, present and stronger; sensory and motor functions, grossly intact
Posterior	No obvious trauma

5. What is the purpose of performing a detailed physical examination?

_____

_____

_____

_____

The patient's condition continues to improve with your treatment. He remains conscious and alert; however, he is still slightly restless. The cardiac monitor displays a sinus tachycardia at 100 beats per minute. With an estimated time of arrival at the trauma center of 10 minutes, you perform an ongoing assessment **(Table 19-5)** and then call your radio report to the receiving facility.

Table 19-5 Ongoing Assessment

Level of Consciousness	Conscious and alert to person, place, and time; slightly restless
Airway and Breathing	Airway remains patent; respirations, 18 breaths/min with adequate tidal volume
Oxygen Saturation	98% (on 100% oxygen)
Blood Pressure	108/70 mm Hg
Pulse	100 beats/min, stronger and regular
ECG	Sinus tachycardia

Upon arriving at the trauma center, you are greeted by the attending physician. After further stabilization in the emergency department, the patient is taken to surgery where a partially severed popliteal artery was found and successfully repaired. Following a brief stay in the hospital, the patient was discharged home.

1. What is the appropriate order of initial management for this patient?

Management for the critically injured patient is based on what is going to kill the patient first. In most cases, airway management takes priority over all else; however, this is not always the case. The following represents the appropriate order of initial management for *this* patient:

- **Bleeding control**
  - The bright red blood spurting from the injury behind the patient's knee suggests a severed or partially severed popliteal artery. If not immediately controlled, severe arterial bleeding can result in death within a matter of minutes.
    - In the case of *this particular patient,* bleeding control takes priority over airway management. Because the patient is screaming in pain, he obviously has a patent airway.

- **100% supplemental oxygen**
  - The patient's respirations, although increased, are producing adequate tidal volume. Therefore, 100% oxygen via nonrebreathing mask is appropriate.
    - This patient is displaying signs of shock (ie, restlessness, tachycardia, diaphoresis). Therefore, 100% supplemental oxygen should be administered as soon as possible.

Monitor the patient for signs of inadequate breathing (eg, shallow depth, decreased mental status) and be prepared to provide ventilatory assistance.

- **Shock management**
  - Elevate the patient's legs 6 to 12 inches.
    - Elevation of the legs will not only help control bleeding from the lower extremity wound, but will facilitate venous return to the right side of the heart (increased preload), increasing cardiac output, and maintaining perfusion to the vital organs of the body.
  - Thermal management
    - Place a blanket on the patient to help maintain body temperature. Patients in shock do not have enough oxygen needed to produce energy and maintain body temperature.
    - Hypothermia interferes with the body's clotting mechanisms and may worsen the patient's bleeding.

2. How will you manage the continued bleeding from the patient's injury?

Initial management for severe bleeding involves applying direct pressure to the wound and elevating the extremity above the level of the heart. Direct pressure and elevation are typically performed simultaneously, and, in the majority of cases, adequately controls the bleeding **(Figure 19-1)**. A pressure dressing should then be applied over the wound to maintain constant pressure **(Figure 19-2)**. If bleeding continues, place additional dressings over the pressure dressing. The site should be closely monitored for signs of continued bleeding, as evidenced by blood soaking through the pressure dressing. The popliteal fossa is a difficult place to secure an adequate pressure dressing. Be prepared to proceed to the next step in bleeding control should direct pressure fail.

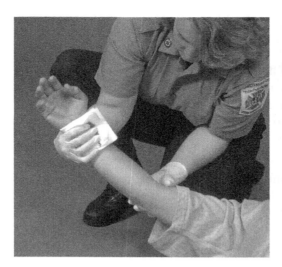

Figure 19-1 Direct pressure and elevation should be performed simultaneously to control severe bleeding.

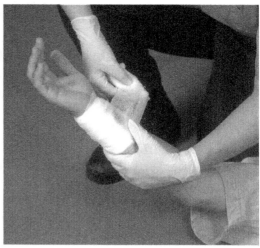

Figure 19-2 Apply a pressure dressing to the wound to maintain constant pressure.

There are occasions when, despite the application of direct pressure, elevation, and pressure dressings, the wound continues to bleed. This is common when large arteries (eg, femoral, radial, popliteal) are damaged or in areas of the body where maintenance of adequate pressure is difficult (eg, popliteal fossa). If, despite initial bleeding control measures, the wound continues to bleed, apply pressure to a proximal arterial pressure point while maintaining direct pressure and elevation **(Figure 19-3)**. Because your patient's injury involves bleeding from the popliteal artery behind the knee, the appropriate proximal arterial pressure point would be the femoral artery. **Figure 19-4** illustrates the major arterial pressure points of the body.

It should be noted that continuing to apply additional dressings to a severely bleeding wound will prove ineffective. Although the blood is contained within the additional dressings, the patient is still losing blood externally. If pressure application at a pressure point proximal to the site of bleeding is ineffective, apply a tourniquet to the extremity proximal to the site of bleeding. This may not be possible if the bleeding is coming from the proximal humerus or proximal thigh—two locations where application of a tourniquet proximal will not be feasible because of the shoulder and hip, respectively. However, for bleeding at the level of the elbow or distal in the upper extremity or at the level of the knee and distal in the lower extremity (as in the current situation), correct tourniquet application is almost always an effective means of controlling bleeding.

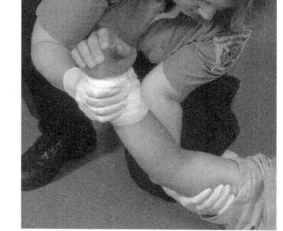

Figure 19-3 If, despite initial efforts to control bleeding, the wound continues to bleed, apply pressure to a proximal arterial pressure point while maintaining direct pressure and elevation.

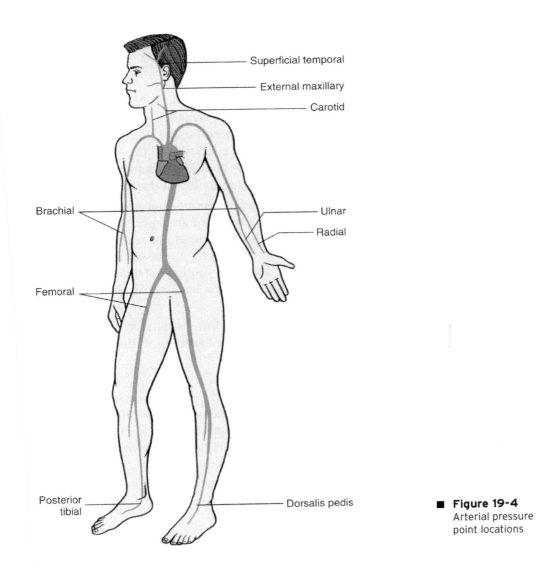

Superficial temporal

External maxillary

Carotid

Brachial

Ulnar

Radial

Femoral

Posterior tibial

Dorsalis pedis

■ **Figure 19-4**
Arterial pressure point locations

Another method for controlling severe bleeding if initial methods fail is to remove all dressings, locate the site of the bleeding, and apply digital (finger) pressure directly to the site. Some EMS system protocols allow the paramedic to clamp the bleeding vessel with a pair of hemostats. In general, this method is less effective than applying pressure to a pressure point and is very difficult to effectively accomplish in the prehospital environment.

In the worst-case scenario, when all attempts to control bleeding fail, immediately transport the patient to the closest hospital while continuing bleeding control efforts en route.

IV therapy would clearly be of no benefit to the patient with severe, uncontrolled bleeding. Remember to focus your efforts on treating what will kill the patient *first*.

3. What is the appropriate IV fluid resuscitation regimen for this patient?

The goal of IV therapy in the shock trauma patient is to maintain adequate perfusion, regardless of whether the patient is bleeding internally or externally. Optimally, lost blood should be replaced with blood. However, because blood must be refrigerated, typed and cross-matched and has a short shelf life, it is not practical for use in the prehospital setting.

Crystalloid solutions, such as normal saline or lactated ringers, are more practical for use in the prehospital setting than blood. They are well-balanced solutions that closely resemble the electrolyte concentration of plasma. Additionally, they are less expensive and have a longer shelf life than blood.

As previously discussed in other case studies within this book, IV therapy for the patient with internal bleeding should be somewhat conservative, infusing just enough IV fluid to maintain adequate perfusion (eg, good mental status, systolic blood pressure of 90 mm Hg). Because internal bleeding cannot be controlled in the prehospital setting, rapid IV fluid infusions may interfere with the body's hemostatic processes, thus resulting in increased internal hemorrhage and deterioration of the patient's condition.

External bleeding, however, can be controlled in the prehospital setting; therefore, IV fluid resuscitation in the hypotensive patient should be more aggressive. After you have controlled all external bleeding and you have no reason to suspect internal hemorrhage, infuse 1,000 mL of a crystalloid solution and then reassess the patient. Continue to administer fluid boluses as needed until you have stabilized the patient's blood pressure at 90 mm Hg and/or systemic perfusion has improved (eg, improved mental status, stronger peripheral pulses).

Because two-thirds of crystalloid solutions leave the intravascular space within 1 hour after administration, you must administer 3 mL of crystalloid solution for every 1 mL of estimated blood loss.

Crystalloid solutions improve tissue perfusion by increasing circulating volume and facilitating the transport of oxygen-carrying red blood cells that remain in the vascular space; however, they do not carry oxygen themselves. Additionally, because excessive crystalloid administration may result in hemodilution of the blood, administration of more than 3 liters in the prehospital setting should be reserved for situations where perfusion cannot be maintained by any other means.

The paramedic should follow locally established protocols or contact medical control as needed regarding IV fluid resuscitation for the shock patient.

4. What is the difference between crystalloid and colloid solutions?

Crystalloid solutions, which are the primary solutions used for prehospital fluid resuscitation, contain electrolytes and water. However, because crystalloids lack proteins and larger molecules, their presence in the vascular space, once administered, is of relatively short duration. Furthermore, crystalloids, unlike whole blood, do not have the ability to carry oxygen.

The three main types of crystalloid solutions are classified by their tonicity (number of particles per unit volume) relative to that of blood plasma:

- **Isotonic crystalloids**
  - Tonicity is equal to that of blood plasma; therefore, in a normally hydrated patient, they will not cause a significant shift in fluids or electrolytes.
  - 0.9% sodium chloride (normal saline) and lactated ringers are examples of isotonic crystalloids.

- **Hypertonic crystalloids**
  - Has a higher solute concentration than that of the cells; therefore, when administered to a normally hydrated patient, they cause fluid to shift out of the intracellular space and into the extracellular space.
  - 50% dextrose in water ($D_{50}W$) is an example of a hypertonic crystalloid.

- Hypotonic crystalloids
  - Has a lower solute concentration than that of the cells; therefore, when administered to a normally hydrated patient, they cause fluid to shift from the extracellular space and into the intracellular space.
  - 0.45% sodium chloride (half normal saline) and 5% dextrose in water (D_5W) are examples of hypotonic crystalloids.

As previously discussed, normal saline and lactated ringers are the most commonly used IV crystalloids in the prehospital setting because of their ability to immediately and rapidly expand circulating volume.

Colloid solutions contain large proteins and molecules that cannot pass through the capillary membrane; therefore, relative to crystalloids, they remain in the vascular space for a longer period of time. Additionally, the osmotic properties of colloids attract water into the vascular space; therefore, a small amount of colloid can significantly increase intravascular volume. The following are examples of colloid solutions:

- **Plasmanate (plasma protein fraction)**
  - The principle protein in plasmanate is albumin, which is suspended in a saline solution.
- **Dextran**
  - Not a protein; however, it contains large sugar molecules with osmotic properties similar to that of albumin.
- **Hetastarch (Hespan)**
  - Similar to dextran in that it contains large sugar molecules with osmotic properties similar to those of proteins
- **Salt-poor albumin**
  - Contains only human albumin. Each gram of albumin administered causes retention of approximately 18 mL of water in the vascular space.

Although colloids maintain vascular volume better than crystalloids, their use in the prehospital setting is not practical. Colloids have a short shelf life, are costly, and have specific storage requirements, attributes that make them more suitable for the hospital setting. Like crystalloids, the colloids listed do not have the ability to carry oxygen.

5. What is the purpose of performing a detailed physical examination?

The detailed physical examination **(Table 19-6)** is a comprehensive head-to-toe examination that is performed on patients who are either critically injured or unconscious. It encompasses all of the components of the initial and rapid assessments; however, it is more in-depth, methodical, and takes more time to perform.

The purpose of the detailed physical examination is to detect injuries or conditions that were either not evident during earlier assessments or that did not require immediate emergency care.

With critically ill or injured patients, you will seldom have time to perform this time-consuming examination because you will often be preoccupied performing ongoing assessments and rendering emergency treatment. If, while en route to the hospital, the patient's condition deteriorates, you should immediately repeat an initial assessment and address any newly developed life-threatening conditions. Because this may occur several times throughout transport, you will likely not have time to perform a detailed physical examination.

If, however, your transport time to the hospital is lengthy and you have addressed all life-threatening injuries or conditions, a detailed physical examination should be performed.

Table 19-6 Detailed Physical Examination

Head
- Inspect and palpate the cranium for bleeding, pain, deformities, or instability.
- Inspect and palpate the facial bones for pain, deformities, or instability.
- Inspect the ears, nose, and mouth for drainage or potential obstructions.
- Inspect the pupils for size, shape, equality, and reactivity to light.

Neck
- Assess the position of the trachea (eg, midline or deviated).
- Inspect the jugular veins for distention.
- Palpate the cervical spine for pain or deformities.

Chest
- Inspect the chest for symmetry, paradoxical movement, retractions, and bruising.
- Palpate the chest for pain, crepitus, or instability.
- Auscultate breaths sounds bilaterally.
  - Determine if breath sounds are equal on both sides of the chest.
  - Note any abnormal breath sounds, such as wheezing, rales, or rhonchi.

Abdomen/pelvis
- Inspect the abdomen for bruising and distention.
- Palpate four quadrants of the abdomen for pain, guarding, rigidity, or masses.
- Palpate the painful area last.
- Palpate the pelvis for pain, crepitus, or instability.
  - Gently push in and down on the iliac crests.
  - Never rock the pelvis back and forth.
  - Do not repalpate the pelvis if it was unstable or painful during previous assessment.

Lower extremities
- Inspect and palpate for pain, crepitus, and deformities.
- Assess gross motor and sensory functions and distal pulses.

Upper extremities
- Inspect and palpate for pain, crepitus, and deformities.
- Assess gross motor and sensory functions and distal pulses.

Posterior
- Inspect and palpate the posterior thorax for pain or deformities.
- Inspect and palpate the lumbar region and buttocks for pain or deformities.
  - Because the patient will often be immobilized on a spine board, you will usually not be able to inspect the posterior in the detailed physical examination.
  - Assessment of the posterior should be performed when you log-roll the patient to place them on the spine board.

It is most appropriate to perform a detailed physical examination of your patient in the back of the ambulance while en route to the hospital. Remaining at the scene to perform a thorough examination on a critically ill or injured patient would clearly delay definitive care and increase the possibility of a poor patient outcome.

Summary

During the initial assessment of your patient, all airway, breathing, and circulation problems must be immediately corrected. Invasive procedures, such as IV therapy or intubation, are of no value to the patient if there is uncontrolled bleeding or a non-patent airway.

The patient in this case study had an obviously patent airway; however, he had an uncontrolled arterial hemorrhage. Therefore, controlling the bleeding had priority over applying oxygen. If, however, sufficient help was available (eg, first responder, law enforcement), then bleeding control and oxygen therapy could have been accomplished simultaneously. Remember that the order in which you manage your patient's injuries or condition is based on what will be the *most rapidly* fatal. A severe, uncontrolled arterial hemorrhage will kill the patient before you can even prefill the reservoir of a nonrebreathing mask!

Once a patent airway has been established and all external bleeding has been controlled, the patient should be rapidly assessed for signs of shock. If signs of shock are present, immediately transport the patient and perform all interventions, such as IV therapy and cardiac monitoring, en route to the hospital.

In addition to 100% oxygen and thermal management, shock caused by external blood loss should be treated with aggressive IV infusions of an isotonic crystalloid solution (eg, normal saline, lactated ringers). The goal of IV therapy is to maintain adequate perfusion (eg, systolic blood pressure of 90 mm Hg, improved mental status). Because crystalloid solutions quickly leave the vascular space, you must infuse 3 mL for each 1 mL of estimated blood loss. Because excessive crystalloids may hemodilute the blood, more than 3 liters should not be administered in the prehospital setting unless absolutely necessary to maintain perfusion.

Continually monitor the patient en route to the hospital and be prepared to infuse additional IV fluids for blood pressure maintenance, assist ventilations for inadequate breathing, or perform CPR if the patient develops cardiac arrest.

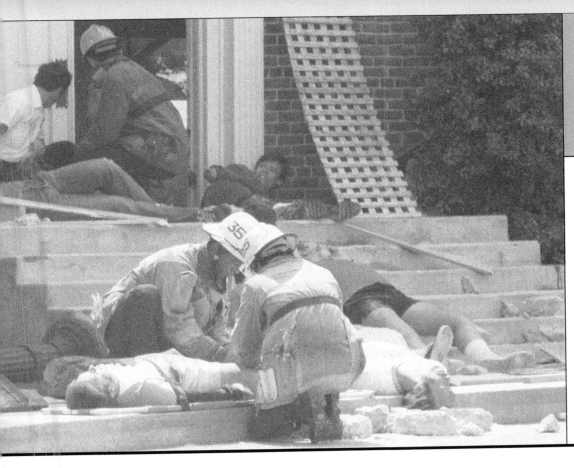

20

A Mass-Casualty Incident

At 1:30 PM, you are dispatched to 115 Main Street, where a car drove off the road and ran into a building. Dispatch advises you that there are four patients. The police department, fire department, and an additional ambulance are immediately dispatched to the scene. Your response time to the scene is approximately 3 minutes.

Your unit and an engine company arrive at the scene at the same time. Law enforcement is providing traffic control. The second ambulance radios you and advises that their response to the scene will be delayed by 7 minutes. You and your partner triage the four patients (Table 20-1). The driver of the car, who refuses EMS care, is being questioned by law enforcement.

Table 20-1 Triage Results

Patient 1: 22-year-old conscious, crying female
- Unable to move her legs
- Abrasions to the face and arms
- Respirations, 20 breaths/min and unlabored
- Pulse, 100 beats/min and strong

Patient 2: 60-year-old conscious, restless male
- Abdominal pain
- Wearing a diabetic bracelet
- Respirations, 24 breaths/min and shallow
- Pulse, 110 beats/min weak and irregular

Patient 3: 41-year-old unconscious male
- Large hematoma to the forehead
- Respirations, 8 breaths/min and irregular
- Pulse, 60 beats/min and bounding

Patient 4: 39-year-old conscious and alert female
- Contusion to the forehead
- Pain in left hip
- Respirations, 22 breaths/min and unlabored
- Pulse, 76 beats/min and strong

1. On the basis of your triage findings, how would you categorize these four patients?

2. What are the components of the START triage system?

You and your partner begin treating the most critically injured patients. You assign fire department personnel, who are certified first responders, to tend to the lesser-injured patients until the second ambulance arrives. You and your partner agree that a third ambulance is needed at the scene.

3. How would you justify the need for a third ambulance?

_____

_____

_____

_____

The second ambulance arrives at the scene, and its crew begins immediate care of the lesser-injured patients. You ask dispatch to notify the local trauma center and advise them of the situation. The dispatcher advises you that the trauma center can accept all four patients.

4. What areas are typically established during a mass casualty incident?

_____

_____

_____

_____

The third ambulance arrives at the scene as you and your partner depart the scene with patient 3. The second ambulance departs the scene shortly thereafter with patient 2. The two lesser-injured patients are cared for and transported to the trauma center by the third ambulance.

CASE STUDY ANSWERS AND SUMMARY

1. On the basis of your triage findings, how would you categorize these four patients?

During mass casualty situations, patients are rapidly triaged and then categorized based on the severity of their injuries or conditions **(Table 20-2)**. The *only* care provided during the triage process is immediate life-saving airway or hemorrhage management. Because the condition of patients may deteriorate, which would require recategorizing them to a different priority (usually higher); triage must be an ongoing process. On the basis of your rapid triage findings, the patients involved in this incident should be categorized as follows:

- **Critical (Red)**: Patients 2 and 3
- **Urgent (Yellow)**: Patients 1 and 4

Patient 2 (red) has signs of shock (ie, tachycardia, tachypnea, restlessness), abdominal pain that is suggestive of intraabdominal bleeding, and an underlying medical history of diabetes, which could exacerbate his condition.

Patient 3 (red) is demonstrating signs of severe head injury. He is unconscious, which places his airway in immediate jeopardy. Additionally, his respirations are 8 and shallow; therefore, he is breathing inadequately.

Patient 1 (yellow) appears hemodynamically stable at present; however, her inability to move her legs suggests a spinal injury. If the mechanism of injury was significant enough to cause spinal injury, she could have also sustained other injuries, which could result in deterioration of her hemodynamic status.

Patient 4 (yellow) is conscious with stable vital signs; however, she is complaining of hip pain, which could indicate a hip fracture. Like patient 1, a mechanism of injury significant enough to cause a high-energy hip fracture could also cause other potentially life-threatening injuries.

Table 20-2 Triage Categories

Critical (Red)
- Patients who need immediate care and transport
  - Airway and breathing compromise
  - Uncontrolled or severe bleeding
  - Altered mental status
  - Severe underlying medical problems
  - Signs of shock (hypoperfusion)
  - Severe burns

Urgent (Yellow)
- Patients whose treatment and transport can be *temporarily* delayed
  - Burns without airway compromise
  - Major or multiple bone or joint injuries
  - Spinal injuries with or without spinal cord involvement

Delayed (Green)
- Patients whose treatment and transport can be delayed until last
  - Minor fractures
  - Minor soft-tissue injuries

Deceased (Black)
- Patients who are already dead or have little chance for survival
  - Cardiopulmonary arrest
  - Injuries that preclude survival (eg, head trauma with exposed brain matter)
  - Signs of obvious death (eg, decapitation, burned beyond recognition)

Because you and your partner are the only two paramedics at the scene, and the arrival of additional ambulances will be delayed, you should begin immediate treatment of the most critically injured patients (patients 2 and 3). Utilize fire personnel to tend to the lesser-injured patients (patients 1 and 4) until additional ambulances arrive.

This incident is classified as a mass casualty incident (MCI). An MCI is defined as any situation that places a great demand on available resources. Clearly, as the sole ambulance at the scene, you and your partner cannot effectively care for all of the patients involved in this incident without assistance.

2. What are the components of the START triage system?

With the START (Simple Triage and Rapid Transport) triage system, a 60-second assessment of each patient is made that focuses on four areas: ability to walk, respiratory rate, pulses/perfusion, and mental status (Table 20-3). The START triage system, which categorizes patients as being delayed (green), urgent (yellow), critical (red), or deceased (black), uses color-coded triage tags to identify the patient's triage category (Figure 20-1).

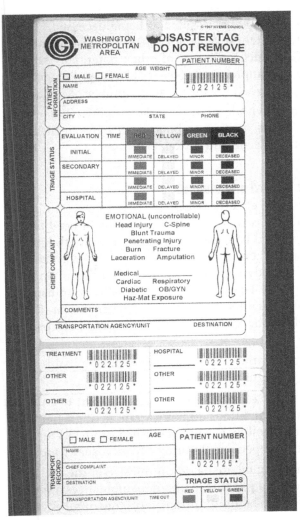
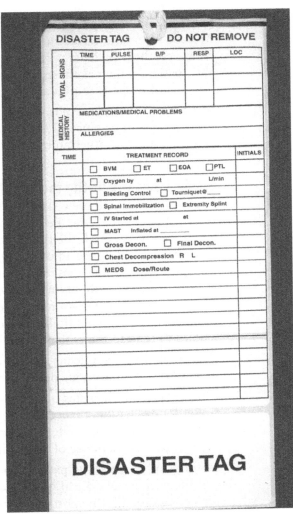

■ **Figure 20-1** A color-coded triage tag

Several different types of triage tags can be used. However, a universally agreed upon color-coding system is used, regardless of the type of triage tag used.

Table 20-3 START Triage System

Able to walk?
- Yes – Delayed
- No – Assess respiratory rate
  - Apneic – Open airway
    - Remains apneic – Deceased
    - Respirations <10 or >30 breaths/min – Critical
    - Respirations >10 but <30 breaths/min – Assess Perfusion
      - Radial pulses absent – Critical
      - Radial pulses present – Assess mental status
        - Follows commands – Delayed
        - Can't follow commands – Critical

Although there are several methods of triage, one commonality is that those who are pulseless or apneic (after opening the airway) are classified as being deceased. Because traumatic cardiac arrest patients rarely survive, focusing your resuscitative efforts on these patients will unnecessarily delay the care of other, potentially salvage-able, patients, such as those with airway compromise or severe bleeding. Remember, the goal of triage is to provide the greatest good for the greatest number of patients.

The START triage system is typically used with large-scale mass casualty incidents; however, it can be a useful system if you are the first ambulance to arrive at the scene and the arrival of other ambulances at the scene will be delayed.

3. How would you justify the need for a third ambulance?

One ambulance and crew (two medics) can effectively care for only one critically injured patient at a time. Because you have two critical patients, you will need two ambulances. Although the two lesser-injured patients (patients 1 and 4) both have the potential for significant injuries (eg, spinal cord injury, hip fracture) and will require transport to a trauma center, they are hemodynamically stable at present and do not require immediate life-saving interventions. Therefore, they could both be transported in the same ambulance—one on the stretcher and the other on the bench seat. If necessary you can assign a firefighter to drive the ambulance, thus allowing both paramedics to tend to the patients.

Because of their significant mechanisms of injury, both patients require spinal immobilization and continuous monitoring for signs of deterioration.

Although the mechanisms of injury of patients 1 and 4 necessitate transport to a trauma center for evaluation, their present clinical conditions do not warrant taking a fourth ambulance out of service. It is important to follow locally established protocols regarding the most efficient use of ambulances and personnel during a mass casualty incident.

Methods of transporting patients to the hospital are based on the size of the incident and the number of critical versus noncritical patients. Although ambulances are the typical method of transportation, buses may be used to transport large numbers of patients categorized as being delayed (green). Aeromedical services should be reserved for transporting critical patients or patients who require resources available only at a trauma center that is a great distance from the scene of the incident.

4. What areas are typically established during a mass casualty incident?

During large-scale mass casualty incidents, responsibilities in eight different areas are assigned by the incident commander. These areas, or sectors, each have their own role in the overall management of the incident. The major areas of a mass casualty incident are as follows:

■ **Command center**
  • The area where the incident commander oversees and coordinates the activities of the other areas.

■ **Staging area**
  • The holding area from where arriving ambulances and crews are assigned particular tasks.

■ **Operations/extrication area**
  • Where patients are disentangled and removed from a hazardous environment, allowing them to be moved to the triage area.

■ **Triage area**
  • A sorting point, which is run by the triage officer. This is where patients are quickly assessed, categorized according to the severity of their injuries, and then, according to their assigned priority, directed to specific locations in the treatment area(s).

■ **Treatment area**
  • Organized and managed by the treatment officer, this area is where a more thorough assessment is made and on-scene treatment is initiated while transport is being arranged.

■ **Supply area**
  • Area where extra supplies and equipment are stored and distributed as needed.

■ **Transportation area**
  • This area, which is managed by the transportation officer, is where ambulances and crews are organized to transport patients from the treatment area to area hospitals.

■ **Rehabilitation area**
  • Provides protection and treatment to on-scene rescue personnel. As personnel enter and exit the scene, they are assessed and provided any needed medical care.

It is crucial that the incident command system remain intact at all times and that all personnel are able to effectively function in each of the eight different areas.

When you arrive at the scene of a mass casualty incident, you will be assigned to a specific area by the incident commander. You should report immediately to that area's officer for further instructions. When you have completed the assigned task, report back to that same officer for another assignment. If your duties in that particular area are complete, you may be reassigned to a different area.

Summary

A mass casualty incident is any situation that overwhelms the available resources of the EMS system, fire department, and area hospitals. Although the word "mass" implies many patients, two critical patients and one ambulance or four noncritical patients and two ambulances are just as much mass casualty incidents as a situation involving 20 or more patients.

This case study presented a relatively small mass casualty incident in which four patients, two of whom were critically injured, were effectively managed by three ambulances. Unfortunately, however, not all incidents are as limited in terms of numbers and criticality of patients.

In large-scale incidents, such as plane crashes, bus wrecks, and building collapses, an EMS system's resources are often quickly depleted and hospitals are quickly filled to capacity. This is when the incident management system is absolutely critical in order to effectively manage the incident and save as many lives as possible.

Once an incident command system has been established, all patients are rapidly triaged and, based on the severity of their injuries, are categorized with color-coded triage tags, which identifies their treatment and transport priority. During the triage process, the only care provided is immediate life-saving airway or hemorrhage management.

Because the patient's conditions may change, triage must be an ongoing process, recategorizing patients as needed. The goal of triage is to provide the greatest good for the greatest number of patients.

Once priority patients are identified, they are sent to the treatment area, where a more in-depth assessment is performed and emergency care is rendered. Following stabilization in the treatment area, patients are then directed by the transport officer to the appropriate medical facility.

The mass casualty incident response that runs the smoothest is one that has been rehearsed. It is important for each EMS system to know its available resources (eg, mutual aid, trauma centers, HazMat teams) and to practice "mock" mass casualty incidents.

Lightning Source UK Ltd.
Milton Keynes UK
UKOW07f1913041016

284433UK00007BA/62/P